Tools and Strategies for the Medical Practice

∾

"Patient Access is essential for healthcare leaders who are responsible for designing and implementing a state-of-the-art patient access management system. Once again, Woodcock and Keegan have distilled the complexities of access management into a practical, must read book. Healthcare consumers equate access with quality and this newly revised version addresses the fact that patient access has moved beyond simple appointment and telephone system management. The book identifies the critical components required to enhance patient access in addition to providing tools, resources, best practices and case studies. It is the roadmap for transformation in patient access management."

CHRISTINE A. SCHON, MPA, MHCDS, FACMPE
Chief Operating Officer
CHESHIRE MEDICAL CENTER / DARTMOUTH HITCHCOCK

∾

"Everyone wants a silver bullet with respect to understanding healthcare patient access and call management. However, these are complicated issues with as many facets as providers who practice within our organizations. Elizabeth and Deborah break down these complications into consumable and manageable parts; providing data points and measures that will guide you on how to make sustainable change."

PAUL SCHMITZ
Director of Patient Access and Capacity Management
PHYSICIAN ENTERPRISE | ADVENTIST HEALTH SYSTEM

∾

"Our healthcare environment demands expertise in finance, technology, strategic planning, marketing, public relations, human resources and operations. However, patient access is the core of our business and is often overlooked. The work of Woodcock and Keegan in this book gives us direction and guidance in developing and managing the critical component of a successful practice…managing patient access, phone procedures and creating a culture of patient first."

PATRICIA L. BREWSTER, MHA, FACMPE
Chief Executive Officer
INTRAHEALTH GROUP AND ORTHOATLANTA

Medical Group Management Association® (MGMA®) publications are intended to provide current and accurate information and are designed to assist readers in becoming more familiar with the subject matter covered. Such publications are distributed with the understanding that MGMA does not render any legal, accounting, or other professional advice that may be construed as specifically applicable to individual situations. No representations or warranties are made concerning the application of legal or other principles discussed by the authors to any specific factual situation, nor is any prediction made concerning how any particular judge, government official, or other person will interpret or apply such principles. Specific factual situations should be discussed with professional advisors

Elizabeth Woodcock & Deborah Walker Keegan, Authors
MGMA (Association); publisher.
EGZ Publications; production.

Woodcock, Elizabeth W.
 Patient Access: Tools and Strategies for the Medical Practice / Elizabeth W. Woodcock, MBA, FACMPE, CPC, Deborah Walker Keegan, PhD, FACMPE.

2nd Edition
(First was "It's Your Call")

Library of Congress Cataloging-in-Publication Data

Names: Woodcock, Elizabeth W., author. | Keegan, Deborah Walker, author. |
 Medical Group Management Association, issuing body.
Title: Patient access : tools and strategies to optimize the medical practice
 / Elizabeth W. Woodcock, Deborah Walker Keegan.
Other titles: It's your call.
Description: Second edition. | Englewood, CO : Medical Group Management
 Association, [2018] | Preceded by It's your call / Elizabeth W. Woodcock,
 Deborah Walker Keegan. c2013.
Identifiers: LCCN 2017034861 (print) | LCCN 2017036004 (ebook) | ISBN
 9781568295343 (e-book) | ISBN 9781568295336 (pbk.)
Subjects: | MESH: Practice Management, Medical--organization & administration
 | Telemedicine | Health Services Accessibility | Telephone | Efficiency,
 Organizational | Communication
Classification: LCC RC480.6 (ebook) | LCC RC480.6 (print) | NLM W 80 | DDC
 362.2/04251--dc23
LC record available at https://lccn.loc.gov/2017034861

Product ID: 9052
ISBN: 978-1-56829-533-6
Production Credits
Senior Product Manager: Craig Wiberg, MLS, MBA
Content Production Manager: Isabel Penraeth, MFA
Senior Content Coordinator: Jody McDonald

Copyright 2018 Medical Group Management Association and Elizabeth W. Woodcock and Deborah Walker Keegan.

All rights reserved. No part of this publication may be reproduced, stored in a retrieval system, or transmitted, in any form or by any means, electronic, mechanical, photocopying, recording, or otherwise, without the prior written permission of the copyright owner.

CPT codes copyright 2018 American Medical Association. All Rights Reserved. CPT is a trademark of the AMA. No fee schedules, basic units, relative values, or related listings are included in CPT. The AMA assumes no liability for the data contained herein. Applicable FARS/DFARS restrictions apply to government use.

Printed in the United States of America
10   9   8   7   6   5   4   3   2   1

Patient Access
Tools and Strategies for the Medical Practice

Elizabeth W. Woodcock, MBA, FACMPE, CPC
Deborah Walker Keegan, PhD, FACMPE

Medical Group Management Association
104 Inverness Terrace East
Englewood, CO 80112-5306
877.275.6462
mgma.com

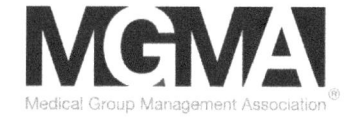

Contents

CHAPTER 1	Overview	1
CHAPTER 2	**Strategy**	3
	Creating a Culture of Access	4
	Balancing Provider Supply and Patient Demand	7
	Optimizing Provider Capacity	8
	Summary	14
CHAPTER 3	**Scheduling Optimization**	15
	Scheduling Methods	15
	Strategies to Optimize Scheduling	17
	Summary	31
CHAPTER 4	**Call Demand and Performance**	33
	Telephones and Quality	34
	Inbound Calls	36
	Outbound Calls	43
	Telephone Quality and Service Expectations	45
	Customer Feedback	52
	Summary	59
CHAPTER 5	**Telephone Access Redesign**	61
	Engage Stakeholders	62
	Telephone Action Plan	63
	Telephone Management—By Call Type	63
	Converting Inbound Calls to Outbound Calls	93
	Reducing Inbound Calls	96
	Summary	101
CHAPTER 6	**Telephone Staffing**	103
	Recruiting Telephone Staff	103
	Creating a Telephone Staffing Model	108

	Staging the Telephones	115
	Staff Education	116
	Staff Resources	118
	Staff Performance Management	119
	Summary	120
CHAPTER 7	**Call Centers**	**123**
	What Is a Call Center?	124
	Key Decision Steps in Call Center Development	127
	Staffing a Call Center	131
	Call Center Design	151
	Summary	158
CHAPTER 8	**Virtual Communication and Telehealth**	**161**
	Patient Portal	163
	Virtual Visits	164
	E-consults	166
	Summary	167
CHAPTER 9	**Communication Tools**	**169**
	Telephone Scripts	170
	Staff Knowledge	177
	Nonverbal Communication Tools	178
	Customer Service Tools	180
	Message-Taking Tools	184
	Callbacks	190
	Summary	198
CHAPTER 10	**Systems and Technology**	**201**
	Voicemail	202
	Automatic Call Distributor	209
	System Selection	214
	Summary	222

CHAPTER 11   Key Performance Indicators ... 223
    Summary ... 229

Conclusion ... 230
Index ... 233
About the Authors ... 237

Acknowledgments

This book is dedicated to the practice administrators, physicians, advanced practice providers, and staff members who manage the patient access challenge in their medical practices day-in and day-out. We are in awe of your tireless efforts to streamline patient and referring physician access, optimize scheduling and improve patient communications.

We also recognize Brent Bizwell of Access Advisors and Roberta Parillo for sharing their insights and lessons learned in call center development.

[CHAPTER 1]

Overview

In this book, we discuss the critical components of patient access and provide tools and resources to help you manage the challenges with this vital aspect of your medical practice.

PROVIDER SUPPLY AND PATIENT DEMAND

Achieving optimal patient access requires a balance of provider supply and patient demand. When these are in imbalance, problematic access abounds. We share strategies to help your practice cultivate a patient access culture and add capacity to your medical practice to help you meet patient demand for services.

SCHEDULING OPTIMIZATION

Optimizing the schedule is one of the critical components of access. If a patient cannot easily obtain an appointment, we are faced with not only a dissatisfied patient, but also considerable rework for medical practice employees. We share scheduling optimization strategies to optimize the provider's time, while at the same time facilitating a streamlined patient flow process.

TELEPHONE MANAGEMENT

Despite the fact the telephone is becoming a dated technology for voice-to-voice exchange, it is the telephone that is ringing off the hook in most medical practices. Telephones have long been a source of frustration for practices and patients alike. Practices struggle to develop the right staffing model, tools and technologies to effectively manage the telephones. On the other hand, patients want their issues addressed immediately and are frustrated with call waiting, messaging and telephone tag. With high volume

– and high expectations – the telephone is an area of the practice that is ripe for opportunity. In this book, we share telephone management tools, staffing and strategies to help you manage your telephones and achieve first call resolution. We also provide a detailed guide to develop and manage a call center or virtual front office for your practice.

VIRTUAL COMMUNICATION AND TELEHEALTH
More and more, patients want to communicate with a medical practice via text and messaging. Many also want to receive care when and where they need it and are increasingly seeking out non-face-to-face encounters like those offered by telehealth and virtual visits. This is a challenge to medical practices as they work to quickly develop their e-clinical and e-business capabilities. We have included a chapter devoted to virtual communication and e-visits to help your practice prepare for these expanded access channels.

KEY PERFORMANCE INDICATORS
We have included key performance indicators (KPIs) and recommended targets for each of these KPIs to help you create a patient access dashboard for your practice. By providing ongoing measurement and monitoring of vital metrics, you can receive early warning of patient access opportunity.

This book gives you the tools and strategies you need to manage the patient access challenge.

CHAPTER 2

Strategy

Many healthcare consumers, including patients, insurers, employers and referring physicians, equate access with quality. It is difficult for a practice to claim to be a high quality provider if patients cannot get appointments. Heightened by provider shortages, increasing numbers of patients with multiple chronic care conditions, and patients' interest in immediate access, medical practices often struggle to determine the best strategic and tactical plans they need to optimize patient access.

Patient access is business-critical for value-based care:

- The Medicare Access and CHIP Reauthorization Act of 2015 (MACRA) Quality Payment Program includes a performance category termed 'improvement activities' that incorporates patient access measures. These measures amplify the focus on patient access.

- With heightened financial accountability for healthcare services, patients are increasingly demanding improved scheduling ease and convenience, along with price transparency. This demand for streamlined velocity to care is a leading factor in the emerging market alternatives, such as retail clinics, urgent care centers, retainer-based practices, and telehealth, with many medical practices working to determine the appropriate strategy to embrace this demand.

- As stakeholders determine the 'best' criteria to measure quality, the relatively simplistic quantification of access—days to next available appointment, for example—has allowed patients, insurers, employers and referring physicians to hone in on access as a key indicator in the healthcare value equation.

Leading access metrics have gained importance in scorecards produced by stakeholders in evaluating medical practices.

Simply having a telephone number—and hoping for the best—will not provide the framework for access success in today's challenging environment. Optimizing patient access requires a strategy, along with tactical plans to meet access targets and goals. In this chapter, we discuss strategic patient access issues, including how to:
- Cultivate an access culture;
- Balance provider supply and patient demand; and
- Optimize provider capacity.

Creating a Culture of Access

Some medical practices are resigned to their current wait times to appointments—and do not perceive the need to operate any differently. Consider these recent conversations:

A urologist stated: 'what is the difference between a 48-hour or 72-hour wait for a patient with an elevated PSA (prostate-specific antigen)?'

A surgeon revealed his lack of motivation to change his wait times, stating that if patients do not want to wait for him, they are welcome to go elsewhere.

A nurse at a multispecialty practice indicated that just because patients think their clinical issues are urgent does not mean that they cannot wait until tomorrow.

Although these statements reflect particular discussions, these sentiments are common. It is true: for some patients, achieving quality outcomes will be no different in a day or two. Thus, attempts to create a target wait time to appointment that is adopted practice-wide can be met with some skepticism. Such a goal, however, helps focus the practice on creating a culture of access.

This culture of access is not exclusively focused on the 'nicety' of patient accommodation. From a business perspective, long wait times to appointments create cadre of patients who are anxious, worried and fearful. These patients consume significant telephone and electronic communication resources of a medical practice, creating an opportunity cost that often adversely impacts the bottom line. In the short-term, the consequences of poor access include nurses and clinical associates focused on high inbound telephone demand; in the long-term, consequences include the potential loss of market share and lost revenue.

The case study, depicted on the following page is a description of a missed opportunity for a patient seeking care at a multidisciplinary practice in the Southeast. This example illustrates how scheduling templates and scheduling rules can get in the way of optimal patient access and business opportunity.

It is clear from this case study that had this established patient been granted a same-day office visit, both the patient and the medical practice would have benefited:

- The patient would have been seen in a timely fashion with streamlined access to care involving internal referrals to imaging and to a specialist within the same multispecialty practice as her primary care physician.
- The practice would have benefited from the significant revenue associated with a primary care office visit, imaging, and the specialist visit and subsequent procedures. Given the imaging and emergency department visit associated with its patient, the practice received a reduction in revenue based on the high cost of this alternative channel of care.

In short, the inability to accommodate a long-standing patient and the scheduling rules and capacity limitations led to a loss for both parties. What is particularly problematic is that the situation would likely have been handled quite differently had the patient's primary care physician been queried in the first place.

> ### ◆ CASE STUDY ◆
>
> THE PATIENT IS AN ESTABLISHED PATIENT OF A PRIMARY CARE PHYSICIAN BASED IN A MULTISPECIALTY PRACTICE RECOGNIZED AS A PATIENT-CENTERED MEDICAL HOME. SHE TELEPHONED HER PRIMARY CARE PHYSICIAN'S OFFICE TO REQUEST AN APPOINTMENT DUE TO ABDOMINAL PAIN. THE PATIENT WAS INFORMED THAT HER PHYSICIAN DID NOT HAVE AN OPEN SLOT TO SEE HER THAT DAY. THE PATIENT THEN ASKED TO SEE ANOTHER PHYSICIAN OR AN ADVANCED PRACTICE PROVIDER IN THE PRACTICE INSTEAD OF HER OWN PHYSICIAN; SHE WAS NOTIFIED THAT NO SAME-DAY APPOINTMENTS FOR HER CONDITION WERE AVAILABLE FROM THESE PROVIDERS. NEEDING TO BE SEEN, SHE THEN PRESENTED TO A RETAIL PHARMACY CLINIC ONLY TO BE TOLD THAT 'ABDOMINAL PAIN' WAS TOO COMPLICATED TO BE SEEN THERE. SHE THEN WENT TO AN URGENT CARE FACILITY; THE PHYSICIAN ORDERED AN ULTRASOUND AND X-RAY. NO DEFINITIVE DIAGNOSIS WAS PROVIDED. RETURNING HOME, HER ABDOMINAL PAIN WORSENED AND THE PATIENT PRESENTED TO THE HOSPITAL EMERGENCY ROOM FOR A FULL WORK-UP.

Importantly, today's patient access challenge often relates to process, not people. Redesigning the process requires more than just another protocol or procedure, however. The computer can offer only so many slots from which to choose; yet, this challenge is arguably not about slots, it's about a culture of accommodation.

While we recognize the provision of care is an art, as well as a science, we've created what amounts to a locked door to the physician. Unlocking that door requires a prescribed step; once inside, the art of taking care of the patient takes over. The question is: can we construct an entranceway that offers more flexibility in how it is unlocked, changing the locking mechanism to benefit both the practice and the patient?

It is not possible to force a shift in perspective. However, if you believe that change can benefit your practice, we recommend using data to build the case for transformation. Capture the following data:

- Lag time—as measured by calendar days, reflective of the patient's perspective—to next available new and established patient appointments.
- Number and type of patients who seek an appointment within a specified timeframe that cannot be accommodated, often referred to as the 'conversion rate.'
- Number and type of these same patients who do not keep their arrived appointment and/or who cancel their appointment prior to being seen, often referred to as the 'scheduled but not arrived rate.'
- Insurer scorecards related to access for which the practice is held accountable pursuant to contract terms or measured against an industry norm.
- Results of the question(s) focused on patient access via the practice's patient satisfaction survey.

A practice's collection of data may be extensive, but the focus is often on charges, revenue and expenses. Indeed, none of these would even exist without a patient first walking through the door. Develop a dashboard of key access metrics based on that which is available and/or can be gathered for a designated period by manual counts. Present these data to practice stakeholders to formulate the current state of access. (See Chapter 11, Key Performance Indicators, for a full discussion of access metrics and targets.)

Balancing Provider Supply and Patient Demand

Fundamentally, optimal patient access requires a balance of provider supply and patient demand. Even if the locking mechanism related to accessing appointments can be altered, supply and demand must be in balance for patients to be accommodated. An imbalance results in an access challenge:

- If there is an insufficient supply of providers to meet current demand; or
- If there is overwhelming patient demand for the current provider supply.

We share methods to measure supply and demand in later chapters, however, for now, it is important to understand this concept of the need to balance supply and demand. When a medical practice is in imbalance, there are only two options: (1) increase provider supply or (2) reduce patient demand.

BEST PRACTICE

DEFINE TARGET LAG TIMES TO APPOINTMENT FOR NEW AND ESTABLISHED PATIENTS. ALSO CONSIDER REFINING THESE TARGETS BASED ON CLINICAL CRITERIA TO ENSURE YOUR PROVIDERS AND SCHEDULERS ARE WORKING IN CONCERT TO MEET PATIENT DEMAND.

Optimizing Provider Capacity

Unlike the manufacturing environment, 'capacity' in healthcare is not well-defined. A hospital may have a better handle on its capacity—the number of beds, operating rooms, and so forth; however, in the ambulatory practice environment it is a significant challenge to understand a practice's current capacity. Capacity, in the ambulatory environment, is defined by time. There is no norm for the capacity of a single physician, and the time spent in seeing patients is challenging to measure and monitor. Generating capacity—additional capacity, that is—requires thoughtful consideration of measuring existing capacity, exploring options to leverage the physician's time in new, innovative ways that may result in more capacity via improved efficiency, recruiting a new provider and/or identifying and resolving barriers related to capacity.

Measuring capacity

Three key measures generally define the provider's capacity in the ambulatory setting: (1) clinic hours per session; (2) number of sessions per week and (3) number of patients the provider can see during that designated time. As an example, let's assume a provider is in clinic 36 hours per week for a total of 45 weeks per year, and has agreed or is contracted to average 4.0 patient visits per hour. The capacity of that provider is 36 hours multiplied by 45 weeks, for a total of 1,620 hours; at 4.0 patient visits per hour, the annual capacity is 6,480 patient visits or 144 visits per week.

Realized utilization of that capacity—often referred to as the 'fill rate'—is of vital importance to understand as actual capacity often differs from perceived capacity. In this example, if this provider averaged 130 patients per week, divide the actual patients seen (130) by the provider's scheduling capacity (144) to arrive at a fill rate of 90.28 percent. Based on our experience, this is a very high fill rate; often, reality is only 60 to 70 percent of the capacity that was thought to be available is filled.

Leave and time-off policies have a significant impact on actual capacity. In some medical practices, a full-time provider may be required to work only 46 weeks per year (with six weeks off for a combination of vacation and continuing medical education), while other medical practices may have more or less time off granted to a full-time provider.

Time off of work is not the only issue; if capacity is focused on the office, other clinical duties may reduce appointment availability. This would include on-call, hospital consults, surgeries and so forth.

To determine capacity for patients seeking appointments in the office, high-performing practices focus on the time that the provider allocates to the office via his or her 'clinic commitment.' This number becomes the basis for comparison against time booked with appointments. The remaining time is then allocated to other duties as appropriate for the provider based on his or her specialty, as well as the expectations of the practice.

In addition to time, protocols adopted by the providers will also have a decided impact on patient access. These may emanate from expectations regarding intra-visit durations, pre-visit testing or perhaps even the provider's preference to see patients with particular complaints or diagnoses. For example, one provider may want to follow-up with patients every two months, while another provider seeing patients with the same diagnosis may deem a six-month follow-up adequate; one physician may require a certain test be ordered by the patient's primary care physician before being seen, while another may not care; finally, one physician may refuse to see a patient with a particular complaint while another physician—even of the same specialty—may accommodate that patient on a same-day basis.

Strive for consensus about protocols among providers, or determine how to identify and address differences without negatively impacting the patient. While there will always be 'exceptions' to the protocols, sharing data, such as frequency of visits per patient who share the same diagnosis, by provider, for example, is a good way to generate discussion among providers.

One of the greatest challenges to patient access is managing patients who have been scheduled, but fail to arrive. In general, these patients fall into three categories: (1) no-shows; (2) cancellations; and (3) bumps. Patients bear the responsibility for no-shows and cancellations. Bumps, on the other hand, are created by providers.

Providers bump patients due to non-preventable reasons (e.g., they are personally ill) or elective reasons (e.g., they have other obligations or priorities). Regardless of the cause, patients who are 'bumped' from their appointment may never return; studies generally find that half of new patients fall into this category. In addition to the high probability of losing that patient, the resources required to manage these bumps—regardless of the reason for them—are monumental. Communicating with patients, determining appropriate dates and times for the rescheduled appointments, and managing established patients' care in the interim, all consume precious resources. Establishing a policy regarding canceling appointments is an important component of a practice's access initiative. High-performers establish a policy to avoid bumps out of convenience, encouraging instead a focus on providers' scheduling leave in an appropriate and timely manner. Often, a timeframe—30 days, for example—is incorporated in the policy for the minimum prior notification period for bumps, coupled with the requirement that patients who are bumped from the schedule for both non-preventable and elective reasons are to be seen within two weeks of the bump (by adding clinics, office hours, or weekend access if necessary).

Migrating to non-face-to-face alternatives

We have tended to view healthcare as an 'if you build it they will come' service with visits held in a building made of bricks and mortar. It is difficult to make the transition from the traditional patient face-to-face visit to other modalities of care. These include clinical outreach, remote monitoring, home care, video and telephonic visits and other similar methods. As the fee-for-service reimbursement focus transitions to value-based reimbursement, these types of modalities are expected to increase patient access. As examples:

- An integrated healthcare system in the Northwest has only a handful of infectious disease (ID) specialists. How can they make do with so few providers? The ID specialists have been tasked with providing immediate consultative services to primary care physicians and see only the most difficult ID patients in a face-to-face visit. The consultations are facilitated by providing an asynchronous communication platform for e-consults via the system's electronic health record system and health information exchange.

- One large surgical practice in the West is working to optimize the surgeons' time in the operating room, delegating many of the preoperative and postoperative visits to other providers, some of which are provided in the patients' homes.

- A multispecialty practice in the South provides telehealth visits for its postoperative patients, saving its providers hours of travel time to remote satellite clinics each week—and enabling its patients to be treated in their own community.

In these examples, the goal has been to extend the limited resource of the provider. They also serve to define a new model of care delivery that is beginning to emerge nationwide as the reimbursement system gets out of the way to permit innovative delivery care models.

Recruiting a new provider

Faced with long wait times to appointment, some medical practices recruit a new provider as part of their access strategy. Before new provider recruitment, make sure your current capacity is optimized. There may be strategic issues that can be addressed to expand capacity. These include:

- Revise the definition of 'full-time' provider and the productivity expectation.
- Define a standard clinic session—for example, 240 minutes—requiring each provider to meet this standard for patient access accommodation.
- Review follow-up visit protocols to determine if modifications are warranted to include replacing face-to-face office visits with a nurse call or home monitoring.
- Review visit types that may be managed by clinical care team members rather than the provider.
- Examine the provider's template to determine if there is any opportunity to improve the slot usage by offering more flexibility in design. (More information about scheduling strategies are in Chapter 3: Scheduling Optimization.)
- Determine if action can be taken to 'clear' the wait time. As an example, if your practice has a wait time to appointment of three weeks today and in one month you still have an appointment wait time of three weeks, your practice is essentially in equilibrium. It may be possible to 'clear' up the wait by holding weekend or extended office hours, thereby getting the practice back to shorter lag times to appointment.

Identifying constraints

In addition to your providers' time, capacity may be constrained by space or staff. Assess opportunities to improve the use of space by determining areas to convert to exam rooms (for example, the area where paper charts were stored), scheduling appointments early in the morning, through lunch and into the evening, or expanding your practice into new space.

Staff can be the most difficult constraint to address, as there is rarely a determination that there are adequate resources. To address opportunities, take time to observe your practice in action for 2 or 3 days, and interview all stakeholders. Contact the manager in another practice (ideally of your same specialty), and compare staffing ratios with him or her, as well as industry normative data for your specialty available from the Medical Group Management Association and/or your specialty association. Staffing a practice is complex; don't make a snap judgement about staff resources, but rather analyze the situation carefully to determine if your workforce is contributing to a capacity constraint.

Before new provider recruitment, make sure your current capacity is optimized by analyzing your existing provider's time, as well as space and staff.

BEST PRACTICE

ANALYZE ACCESS AND PRODUCTIVITY IN COMBINATION. CREATE A TWO-BY-TWO CHART WITH THE X-AXIS THE AVERAGE APPOINTMENT LAG TIME FOR NEW PATIENTS IN CALENDAR DAYS AND THE Y-AXIS PHYSICIAN WORK RELATIVE VALUE UNITS PER DAY IN COMPARISON TO INDUSTRY BENCHMARK OR INTERNAL MEDIANS. PLOT EACH PROVIDER IN THE PRACTICE TO DETERMINE IF THERE ARE PROVIDER OUTLIERS WHO MAY BENEFIT FROM CHANGES TO THEIR SCHEDULING TEMPLATE, CLINICAL MENTORING OR OTHER MEASURES. SUCH A PRODUCTIVITY/ACCESS GRID IS A RELATIVELY SIMPLE WAY TO GET ANSWERS TO THE COMPLEX QUESTIONS OF IF AND WHEN TO RECRUIT A NEW PROVIDER TO THE PRACTICE.

Summary

Once you have developed a patient access strategy—to include cultivating an access culture, balancing provider supply with patient demand and optimizing capacity—and have defined the access goals for your medical practice, you are in an excellent position to develop the tactical plans to achieve that vision. Tactical plans for performance improvement in patient access include scheduling optimization, telephone call management, virtual communication and telehealth. Chapters in this book are devoted to each of these tactics.

[CHAPTER 3]

Scheduling Optimization

A key tactical element for successful patient access is the ease and timeliness of scheduling an appointment. The scheduling methods embraced by a medical practice have an obvious impact on the efficiency and effectiveness of patient access.

In this chapter, we discuss:

- Scheduling methods; and
- Scheduling optimization strategies.

Scheduling Methods

There are three basic scheduling methods: single interval, modified wave, and advanced access.

Single interval scheduling

Single interval scheduling is the traditional way visits have been scheduled. Each patient is appointed to the template based on a specific time duration. As an example, patients are scheduled into a 15-minute slot or a 30-minute slot based on their appointment type or chief complaint. Slots may vary based on new versus established patient status and/or complexity, such as a post-hospital discharge encounter versus an acute problem such as a runny nose and fever.

Some medical practices have adopted a variation on the single interval scheduling method by offering only one appointment duration for all patients. Instead of struggling to determine the correct time duration needed for a patient visit, all patients are booked into a standard time slot.

As an example, regardless of the reason for visit, the patient is given a 20-minute slot. With this approach, there may be portions of the day when a provider is behind or ahead of schedule, however, in general, the provider catches up by the end of the session. For a provider with eight hours of patient access time, a standard 20-minute slot translates to capacity for 24 patients per day. It is still too early to tell if this approach will be adopted industry-wide, however, it is worth careful consideration, particularly if you already experience a discrepancy between the time slot in which the patient is scheduled and your actual visit times.

Modified wave scheduling

As an alternative to single interval scheduling, modified wave scheduling clusters patients at the beginning of the hour, with the appointments tapering off as the hour concludes. As an example, if the visit interval is 15 minutes for each appointment, four patients (or more to anticipate no-shows and cancellations) are scheduled at the top of the hour. This permits patients to be roomed and ready for providers as it mitigates the issues associated with a visit concluding early or a late-arriving patient.

Advanced access scheduling

The third and most sophisticated of the scheduling methods, advanced access scheduling is the easiest scheduling method from a scheduler's perspective. It permits patients 'to be seen when they want to be seen.' In this scheduling method, some new patient visits and follow-up patient visits are pre-scheduled, however, much of the provider's daily template is open. When patients contact the practice for a same-day appointment, the patient is slotted into an open visit slot. At the beginning of the day the scheduling template may look to be only 20 percent full, however, by the end of the day the provider may have seen patients up to his or her full capacity. A key advantage of this scheduling method is patients are readily granted same day or next day access and there is minimal rescheduling or no-shows to manage.

Strategies to Optimize Scheduling

There are a variety of tools that can be used to optimize scheduling to enhance access. We encourage you to evaluate each of the following scheduling techniques for your medical practice.

Reduce scheduling complexity

When patient visit slots are identified by specific diagnosis or type of visit, the scheduling templates become overly complex. Rather than have 20 different scheduling types, consider a more simplistic approach with the recognition that the often-extraordinary time spent in assessing the specific circumstances for the patient does not result in accuracy of predicting the specific visit time. In sum, determining the specific time in advance of the appointment is quite time-consuming and often fails to serve its purpose. Therefore, practices have realized that basic groupings–like 'short', 'long' and 'procedure'–provide a framework for success that minimizes the time involved in the scheduling process while still allowing for sufficient time on the schedule. This simplicity can improve access for patients and optimize the provider's time.

Reduce barriers

Even if the slots are allocated in an effective manner, the rules of appointing often get in the way. Having been chastised before for scheduling the 'wrong' patient, schedulers become hesitant. Others have just been told not to schedule without permission.

Once the templates are defined, let the schedulers schedule. Do not require the schedulers to take messages for the clinical team for a same-day add-on appointment. Instead, define the criteria schedulers are to use to make scheduling determinations without the need to interrupt the care team simply to schedule a patient for an appointment. The goal should be to accommodate patients, not devote significant resources in deflecting patient demand.

> **BEST PRACTICE**
>
> LET THE SCHEDULER'S SCHEDULE! THE GOAL SHOULD BE TO ACCOMMODATE PATIENTS, NOT DEVOTE SIGNIFICANT RESOURCES TO DEFLECTING PATIENT DEMAND.

Start on time

The construct of most practice management systems is to establish a daily schedule for each provider. The key question to ask is 'who is the schedule for?' Is the schedule for the patient, the clinical support staff or the provider? Each of these individuals often erroneously interpret the schedule for themselves. As an example, if a patient is given a 10:00 a.m. appointment time, that patient expects to be seen by the provider at that time. The nurse, medical assistant or technician may regard the time as that which is for rooming and clinical intake. Similarly, a provider who views the same schedule may assume that the patient slotted for 10:00 a.m. will be roomed and ready by that stated time. This incongruence causes frustration by patients, staff and providers alike.

Discuss this dichotomy with your providers and clinical support staff and create realistic expectations regarding the 'roomed and ready' timeline. If you decide the daily schedule is for the provider, require the schedulers to cite an 'arrival' patient time 10 to 20 minutes prior to the visit so that the patient can be roomed and ready. If the decision is made that the schedule is for the patient, build in a 10-minute lag when viewing the schedule and utilize this new time to identify if the provider is running on time for the day.

To ensure that each clinic session starts on time, give the patients scheduled in the first appointment slots of the morning and the first appointment slots of the afternoon arrival times to correspond with the actual clinical preparation for the visit. As an example, a patient scheduled for an 8:00 a.m. visit should be given an appointment arrival time of 7:40 a.m. to ensure the patient is roomed and ready for the visit. Adopt this same approach for the first slot in the afternoon. This will help each clinic session to start on time and minimize scheduling delays.

There is no single strategy to deploy, as every practice maintains a unique workflow. The key is to understand yours, and establish a protocol to allow the office schedule to truly start—and stay - on time.

Deploy strategic booking

Given the fact that there are multiple stages related to the patient's visit, there is opportunity to engage in strategic booking of appointments. At minimum, we recommend strategic overbooking to manage two common, recurring issues:

- No-shows and cancellations. Schedule in anticipation of no-shows and same day cancellations. As an example, if a provider who has capacity for 24 visits per day has a 10 percent no-show rate, schedule an additional 2 or 3 visits to ensure that the provider's capacity is equal to the provider's arrived patient volume. Or, if there is an opportunity to predict a no-show—for example, a post-ED visit with a 24-year-old male, uninsured patient—then double book that slot. This approach allows the provision of a designated appointment for the patient, while mitigating the risk to the practice related to the loss of the provider's time if the patient fails to show.

- Clinical support staff preparation. Your clinical support staff room the patient, take vitals, take medical and social history, and may obtain specimens, draft orders, etc. in anticipation of the visit. Patients often must travel to the restroom, laboratory, or spend time in undressing. Depending on your specialty and clinical protocols, this typically consumes 5 to 15 minutes.

Recognize this time spent by non-providers in preparation for the visit by strategically double-booking multiple slots per day. This typically involves scheduling a long or complicated visit at the same time as a visit of shorter duration. The strategic double-booking allows the provider to see the patient with the short visit while the clinical assistant conducts the preparation needed for the patient who has the long visit. As an example, schedule a well-woman physical at the same time as a patient who complains about a rash, with both visits scheduled at 9:00 a.m. The clinical assistant first rooms the short visit and while the provider is in the exam room seeing that patient, the clinical assistant is rooming and preparing the patient for the long visit. The provider can seamlessly move from the short visit to the long visit in this fashion.

BEST PRACTICE

TO OPTIMIZE THE PROVIDER'S TIME, SCHEDULE A LONG OR COMPLICATED VISIT AT THE SAME TIME AS A VISIT OF SHORTER DURATION. THIS STRATEGIC OVERBOOKING ALLOWS THE PROVIDER TO SEE THE PATIENT WITH THE SHORT VISIT WHILE THE CLINICAL ASSISTANT CONDUCTS THE PREPARATION NEEDED FOR THE PATIENT WHO HAS THE LONG VISIT.

Establish a target wait time to appointment

Determine a goal for the wait time to new appointment, for example, 72 hours or 14 calendar days, and measure and monitor this data. Proactively establishing an approach to appointment availability allows you to maintain growth in your practice. If your practice can accommodate this target time, consider establishing a guarantee of availability. Marketing your practice's wait time can differentiate your practice and help grow market share, while ensuring timely access to patients.

Standardize and stagger clinic sessions

Establish a standard approach to each half-day clinic session, which permits the most effective staffing. For practices with multiple providers, consider staggering some of the providers' start and stop times within each clinic half-day session to facilitate a natural wave approach to patients' arrivals. This may reduce the likelihood of boluses of patients, that often devolves into long waits and delays. Furthermore, a staggered approach may enhance the opportunity to utilize space effectively. As an example, some providers will have a morning session that starts at 8:00 a.m. with the last patient scheduled at 11:30 a.m., others will commence at 8:15 a.m. and conclude with an 11:45 a.m. appointment, and still others will begin at 8:30 a.m. with a final 12:00 noon appointment slot. The standardized hours per clinic session optimizes patient access and the staggering of the session start and stop times reduces variation in arrival and departure times in the clinic, thereby improving patient flow and service. Of course, staffing patterns need to appropriately align with the schedule.

Target patient visit volume

Create specialty-specific targets for patient visit volume per half-day clinic session. As part of this process, create goals for new patient volume. Track and trend this information monthly to identify opportunities related to clinic session assignment and market share growth. Recognize that incentives around work relative value units (wRVUs) may not be effective. Although pace varies between physicians, most have a lower output of wRVUs per minute of time seeing new patients, in contrast to established patients.

BEST PRACTICE

INCENTIVES INVOLVING WORK RELATIVE VALUE UNITS (wRVUs) WON'T GET THE JOB DONE; ALTHOUGH PACE VARIES BY PHYSICIAN, MOST HAVE A LOWER OUTPUT OF wRVUs PER MINUTE OF TIME SEEING NEW PATIENTS IN CONTRAST TO ESTABLISHED PATIENTS THUS MAKING THEM LESS LIKELY TO SEE NEW PATIENTS IF MOTIVATED BY wRVU PRODUCTION.

Educate clinical staff to scheduling
Make sure clinical support staff know how to schedule patient appointments. When nurses or medical assistants are speaking with a patient and an appointment is required or a change to the schedule is necessitated, these staff should be trained to schedule a patient. This transaction should occur at the time of the telephone triage call rather than require a transfer of the caller to a scheduler.

Predict demand
Integrate analytical tools to improve the practice's business intelligence regarding appointments. Predictive analytics can be used to anticipate patient demand. As an example, one can anticipate the number of hospital follow-up slots that are needed based on patient discharges. Alternatively, predictions can be made based on patient admissions. As another example, the panel size of a provider can be used to determine the number of appointment requests that will be received each day. For greater accuracy, the panel should be adjusted for gender, age and insurance coverage.

Evaluate space
Medical practices invest in space that is available 24 hours a day, seven days a week. However, the facility is only used for a portion of that time. This facility utilization level is further eroded by providers who are assigned exclusive access to a designated area, work part-time, do not hold office hours on a particular day or session of the week, or truncate the number of hours they work. Finally, a significant portion of the space is dedicated to waiting areas.

Particularly if space is a constraint, this is an opportune time to evaluate the use of your space. Avoid assigning exam rooms, instead allowing use by any provider. Share space among part-timers and those who are not in the office every or all day, coordinating schedules to optimize the use of the space. Determine any space that can be converted to exam rooms, to include space that was formerly dedicated to the storage of paper charts.

Level load

Requests for appointments are naturally higher on Mondays, given the fact that there is pent-up demand from the weekend. This same phenomenon of 'spikes' in demand may occur on another day of the week, in the event a provider is out of the office. For example, a surgeon who is in the operating room on Tuesday and Wednesday may experience heightened demand on Thursday. This same infusion of demand occurs seasonally as well. The fluctuation in volume creates boluses of work for the office, yet the number of exam rooms and staff remains consistent. The problem has become so acute that many practices shut down on Fridays to 'prepare' for Mondays.

The concept of level loading the schedule involves balancing patient demand and provider supply. Although there is a portion of patient demand that cannot be anticipated—for example, a patient who becomes ill overnight and needs to be seen acutely the following morning—there is a significant percentage of demand that can be controlled. This is in the form of follow-up visits. If demand for acute appointments is higher on Mondays, then reduce the volume of follow-up appointments that are scheduled on Mondays.

Depending on the specialty of your medical practice and/or its geographic location, you may experience fluctuations in patient demand based on seasonality. As an example, orthopaedic practices located in winter ski resort areas and primary care practices located near destination vacation spots will likely experience a seasonality dimension. Similarly, flu season and the need for back-to-school physicals may cause seasonal peaks in demand for your services.

Evaluate data by recording the number of patients seen each week over the past year. Determine if you have a predictable pattern of demand, which can provide guidance in anticipating the subsequent cycle of higher-than-average demand. If you do have seasonal patterns, create additional capacity to meet this demand. Note that this can be a short-term strategy, for example, offering early morning walk-in clinics only during flu season, or it may lead to decisions to more permanently alter provider schedules to include re-evaluation of time-off, potential for 'provider-of-the-day' models and others. The key is to proactively analyze and plan for these fluctuations in patient demand.

Consider also the opportunity to flex staff to meet the influx of work necessitated by times of heightened patient demand. As an example, this may involve scheduling employees for a 10-hour shift on Mondays, hiring a part-time employee to work on Monday and Tuesday, or contracting with per-diem staff to work during the winter.

Refine this analysis by clinic hour. Morning hours are often fully scheduled, with late afternoon hours lightly scheduled. Patients begin to get backed up by mid-morning rather than be smoothly managed across the day. Strive to level load your day—consider 'starting' patients 15 to 20 minute earlier in the day so that the mid-morning crunch is avoided.

Work to standardize the number of patients to smooth demand, matched with the number of providers to provide a consistent capacity, thus alleviating the influx of patients on certain days and times that overwhelm supply. Although a perfectly even level will not be achieved on a consistent basis, striving for a relatively steady volume equates to the best use of allocated resources and improves patient access and experience.

Cluster diagnoses
Schedule patients with a similar diagnosis in 'clusters' if efficiencies can be gained without an adverse impact on patient access or experience. These may occur during a certain hour, or certain days of the week. This permits the practice to streamline patient flow by ensuring an optimal rhythm and tempo for providers and clinical support staff to manage these patients, gaining efficiency and speed through repetitive services and work processes. For example, postoperative visits, antepartum visits, school physicals and many other types of visits are appropriate candidates to cluster to gain efficiencies by using the same processes, supplies, equipment, and often, mindset.

Clustering is also advantageous for multidisciplinary clinics, such as for transplant patients and oncology patients that involve multiple care team members and/or combinations of visits and treatments on the same day. Coordinate these appointments during the same visit, or within a designated timeframe. This is commonly referred to as 'complex scheduling' or 'itinerary-based scheduling.' This coordinated appointment process not only ensures patient convenience, but also facilitates clinical communication among care team members regarding the patient's care and treatment.

Reduce backlogs

Specific techniques can assist in managing backlogs in the schedule and reducing long lag times to appointments. These include:

- Look forward on the schedule. Contact patients whose appointments are several weeks into the future and accommodate them via expanded hours, additional clinics, weekend clinics, or e-visits, if appropriate.

- Conduct a daily sweep. Each afternoon, look at tomorrow's schedule for openings. These may be a result of patient cancellations or changes to the provider's schedule. Regardless of the reason, look for openings that can be filled. Communicate with patients who are scheduled in the future to determine the opportunity to appoint them for the following day. Proactively maintaining a waitlist (also referred to as a priority list) allows this process to be performed seamlessly. Automate the process, if the opportunity allows.

- 'Max pack' the visit. Pull work into the day. For example, if the patient has a same-day visit, as well as an upcoming physical, consider conducting the physical now rather than delay this service. This provides a great experience for the patient (who is less inconvenienced by having to travel to the practice twice), and also results in opening up a visit slot to accommodate another patient.

- Delegate visits to members of the care team. Use advanced practice providers and nurses to the top of their licensure.
- Assess patient graduation. Evaluate patients to determine if they can be transitioned or graduated back to their primary care physician for routine issues or for continued follow-up care. Some medical specialists, such as cardiologists, for example, may find that over time they are seeing patients for each of their internal medicine needs, rather than co-managing the patient with the patient's primary care provider.
- Conduct outreach care management. Evaluate patients to determine if they need a face-to-face visit or if an outreach call with a member of the care team, home monitoring, telehealth, or a home visit may be clinically appropriate in lieu of a face-to-face office visit.

Manage last-minute cancellations

Develop protocols to manage last-minute cancellations to expand patient access to your practice and fill these critical visit slots. Consider these tactics to handle last-minute cancellations effectively.

- Work your priority list. Maintain a priority list (a priority list is a wait list with a name that invokes importance) of patients who seek to be seen prior to their original appointment date and time.
- Query open orders. If a patient was asked to schedule a future appointment, for example, a six-month follow-up appointment and it is not yet scheduled, proactively contact the patient to schedule the appointment.
- Target patients with chronic disease. Evaluate the records of your chronic disease patients and ensure they have been seen within your recommended timeframe; query the orders database to make sure patients have received the recommended screening, testing or specialty consultations. If they have not yet received them, reach out to the patient to schedule these visits.

Deploy group visits

Medical practices have embraced group visits for cohorts of patients who require in-depth education, informational data and/or involve multiple care team members. A group visit permits providers to see six to twelve patients at once. Instead of a traditional 20-minute encounter with one patient, a provider can see a group of patients in just 60 to 75 minutes. Rather than repeating educational or informational data with each patient, a group visit permits the provider to share this information one time with the group, with each patient seeing each member of the care team individually as appropriate for that patient, and the patient's condition.

Evaluate your patients and identify if there is a significant cohort of patients with a similar diagnosis that may benefit from this streamlined access method. As an example, patients with asthma, diabetes, arthritis, chronic obstructive pulmonary disease or chronic headaches, to name a few, may be candidates for group visits. Similarly, obstetrical patients or nine-month well-child visits may be candidates for group visits in your practice. Ask patients if they are interested in such an option and ensure appropriate confidentiality waiver agreements are in place to protect participating patients. Some patients may welcome a group visit, particularly if this allows an environment to share with patients experiencing similar challenges and gives them quicker access to their provider.

Extend hours

Evaluate your office hours and determine if they are meeting patient demand. It may be that patients are seeking alternative hours, such as the following:

- Same-day urgent care;
- Early morning walk-in;
- Evening walk-in and/or scheduled appointments;
- Weekend walk-in and/or scheduled appointments; or
- Lunch-time appointments.

Time-starved patients benefit from hours outside of the traditional 9:00 a.m. to 5:00 p.m., particularly because this same time coincides with their workday.

Manage no-shows

Our research shows that, in general, 8 percent of scheduled patients fail to keep their appointment. Moreover, all indications are that the frequency of patients missing their scheduled appointment is likely to increase, particularly with the shifting financial burden of healthcare to the patient. The impact to a practice's bottom line is obvious when patients fail to keep their scheduled appointments in terms of lost revenue and unused fixed costs.

To ensure that your no-show patients do not further erode patient access opportunity in your medical practice:

- Do not give frequent no-show patients 'prime' appointment slots. Schedule potential no-show patients during lunch or at the end of the day so they do not artificially block access opportunity to other patients.

- Consider charging fees for no-show appointments to minimize no-shows. Note that such a policy requires an advance notification to patients. Also, fees must be reasonably determined and assessed fairly. Further, patient collection processes must be determined before implementing such a policy. Consider an assessment after the second or third no-show, or collect the patient's credit card in advance (after consulting with an attorney to determine the legality of this based on your services, participation agreements, as well as local and state laws).

- Improve appointment lag time. When patients can access an appointment quickly, they are more likely to keep their appointments. Patients who are scheduled far out into the future may 'shop' for earlier care—or simply get better on their own - and may not contact your practice to cancel their scheduled appointment.

- Remind patients of their appointments via multiple technologies. For example, supplement (or replace) your electronic telephonic reminder confirmation protocols with texting or portal-based notifications. Additionally, for long visits, make a 'warm' confirmation call (from a real person).

- Make it easy for patients to cancel. Rather than require patients to contact you during office hours to cancel a scheduled appointment, offer 24-hour, 7 days a week access to a cancellation e-mail, portal-based notification or telephone number. Also begin to track the timing of appointment scheduling and patient cancellation to guide future scheduling protocols.

- Standardize no-show follow-up. The clinical team should guide the next step to be taken for no-show patients. This may include contacting the patient, rescheduling the patient's appointment, or taking another action. Document all follow-up actions in the patient's medical record. Patients who frequently no-show should be evaluated for dismissal from the practice. Discuss your protocols for dismissing patients with your malpractice carrier, establish your guidelines in writing and ensure they are consistently applied.

- Deploy self-scheduling to allow your patients to choose appointment dates and times. Allow access to self-scheduling 24 hours a day, 7 days a week.

Recall patients

Patients who are scheduled far in advance have a high probability of failing to keep their appointment. Our research shows that the 'tipping point' is 12 weeks; that is, half (or more) established patients who are scheduled for a follow-up visit more than 12 weeks into the future do not keep their appointment as scheduled. These patients will typically contact the practice to reschedule the visit, cancel their appointment, fail to keep their appointment (no-show), or the visit is often bumped by the provider. The schedule thus may look to be full, however, there is additional capacity as the time to the appointment nears.

Calculate the percentage of your 'scheduled but not arrived patients,' to include the categories of no-show, cancellations, bumps and other reasons, comparing this with the lag time to appointment. If you find, for example, that patients who are scheduled more than 12 weeks into the future constitute a higher percentage of scheduled but not arrived patients, consider utilizing a recall system rather than a long scheduling horizon.

Recall is a term used to identify an approximate timeframe for a patient for a follow-up appointment. The date and time are not provided, however, a notification is sent to the patient approximately four weeks in advance to schedule the appointment in the prescribed timeframe. A recall is, in essence, a prescription for an appointment; the specific date and time are decided upon just a few weeks in advance.

Although 12 weeks may be a target date to switch from appointing to recalling, some practices find a need to recall at six weeks—while others consider 18 weeks appropriate. This timeframe is referred to as your 'scheduling horizon,' and can vary by practice and even by provider within a practice. It is best to be consistent with your approach so that your support staff knows when to appoint the patient or when to recall instead.

Most practice management systems permit an electronic recall option to identify the next visit that the provider has recommended for the patient, such as follow-up visit or procedure. If this is not available to your medical practice, consider stand-alone registries as part of an electronic health record (EHR) system or build the functionality into your patient portal. As an alternative, manual or electronic logs, paper or electronic calendars or even a file card system are adequate. Regardless of how you structure your recall system, it can be a valuable tool to facilitate timely patient access, reduce 'holes' in the schedule, and prevent the rework associated with changes to the schedule.

> **BEST PRACTICE**
>
> DO NOT SCHEDULE PATIENTS OUT BEYOND A 12-WEEK PERIOD. INSTEAD, UTILIZE TECHNOLOGY TO RECALL PATIENTS FOR APPOINTMENTS. THIS REDUCES RESCHEDULING, NO-SHOWS, CANCELLATIONS AND PROVIDER BUMPS.

Keep a priority list

Maintain a list of patients who seek to be seen earlier than their current appointment. This will help you fill cancelled visits. The priority list can be maintained in a spreadsheet file if such functionality is not built into your practice management system. In addition to the patient's cellular telephone number, include the date the patient is placed on the list and when the appointment is scheduled so the list can be updated. Highlight the names of all patients who are accommodated and be sure employees close the loop by releasing those patients' originally scheduled appointments.

Summary

These strategies are designed to improve the timeliness and ease with which patients and referring physicians access your practice, while also optimizing the provider's time. Evaluate each of these scheduling methods and optimization strategies for your medical practice. The provider's time is not only a finite resource, but also the most important resource a medical practice has to offer.

CHAPTER 4

Call Demand and Performance

The telephones are the main driver of patient access and are the window through which patients first view your practice. Yet only recently have they been recognized for the role they play in helping—or hindering—patient access. Historically, there was little reason to focus on patient-practice communication; patients were not only very accommodating, but physician schedules were so full that medical practices had no need to improve patient access.

Times have changed. Today's medical practices cannot afford to overlook the important role telephones play in the success of a medical practice. Consider this: the telephone is your physicians' main link to the community. Without it, patients don't get scheduled, referrals are not made or received, triage is delayed or doesn't happen, after-hours questions from patients are late or don't get handled, prescriptions don't get renewed, and claims can't be followed up. The telephone also impacts the financial viability of a medical practice; over the telephone, we learn the patient's demographic and insurance information to permit billing for rendered services, obtain required referrals, and determine what payment to collect from the patient at the point of care. Not only do telephones affect each of these processes, but they are also the patient's first impression of your practice. Historically all but ignored, telephones are a core operational process that defines your level of customer service.

The telephone is a critical access point that requires appropriate staffing and management to provide value—high quality at low cost. Indeed, in some medical practices, more care is provided and/or coordinated via the telephone than ever before. Nurse triage and advice, case management, health coaching, patient navigation, and telehealth are expanding to provide patients with new access channels for care. In addition, patient expectations regarding service and turnaround times associated with the telephones are heightened, with patients requesting answers to their questions now. Gone are the days of patients telephoning the practice and being transferred directly to voicemail, which is checked only a few times during the day. Your patients expect timely and informed responses each and every time they call or message your practice.

Telephones and Quality

It is important to recognize the role telephones play in ensuring high-quality patient care. An overlooked telephone message, a message taken that is incomplete or erroneous, or a lack of due diligence in oral communications with the patient, all may lead to serious complications—and potential malpractice risk. The telephones need to be managed and staffed with the same careful attention as you manage the face-to-face visit with the patient.

Most medical practices have anecdotal data regarding their telephone access. For example, patients complain about busy signals or long hold times, and referring physicians voice concerns that they can never get through on the telephone. At the same time, employees spend an inordinate amount of time picking up voicemail, taking messages, or calming patients who have called multiple times without receiving a response. From a pesky operational issue that always seems broken to a quality-of-care issue that results in a malpractice case, the anecdotes help us see that our telephones are broken, but they do little to assist us in identifying the root cause of the problem and taking appropriate action to resolve telephone problems.

In this chapter, we show you how to convert anecdotes to data by measuring the current call demand and the performance of your telephone processes. This gives you the data needed to evaluate the

[CHAPTER 4] | CALL DEMAND AND PERFORMANCE

root cause of telephone problems and guide you in redesigning your telephone processes and creating an action plan for improvement.

In this chapter, you learn to:

- Determine inbound telephone call volume;
- Measure the reasons for inbound telephone calls;
- Monitor telephone quality; and
- Create telephone service expectations.

BEST PRACTICE

MEASURE YOUR KEY TELEPHONE PERFORMANCE MEASURES—BOTH VOLUME AND QUALITY—TO DETERMINE PATIENT ACCESS OPPORTUNITIES FOR YOUR MEDICAL PRACTICE.

To effectively manage your telephones, you need to achieve the right balance of volume and quality. Let's assume there is no change to your current telephone operations. If call volume increases, quality will typically fall, as your employees are asked to manage a higher volume of work. Similarly, if your expectations for quality are lowered, your practice can manage a higher call volume. Therefore, you need the right balance of volume and quality to optimize telephone patient access to your practice. This chapter commences with a section focused on volume, followed by a detailed discussion of quality metrics.

Before moving ahead with any major modifications in how you manage your telephone system or purchase upgrades to the system's hardware or software, measure your telephones in three areas: (1) call volume, (2) reasons for inbound calls, and (3) quality. The measurements play a dual role: they give you information regarding the performance of the current state of your telephones and they help you measure the impact of changes you make as you improve telephone management in your practice.

BEST PRACTICE

YOU NEED TO ACHIEVE THE RIGHT BALANCE OF VOLUME AND QUALITY TO OPTIMIZE TELEPHONE MANAGEMENT.

Inbound Calls

The first step is to capture the volume of inbound calls received by your medical practice. Determine the following data:

1. Inbound call volume by day of week
2. Inbound call volume by time of day

There are two ways to capture this data—electronically or manually. To capture the inbound call volume electronically, consult with your telephone system vendor to learn what data reports it is able to provide. How to access the system's reporting information may also be outlined in your telephone system's instruction manual. Modern systems should be able to produce reports regarding call volume. You can also invest in reporting software that integrates with your telephone system and monitors these important statistics. Also, when buying your next telephone system, consider only those that put performance indicators and reporting capabilities at your fingertips.

If your telephone system does not report the data, do not dismay. You can still obtain information through manual tracking efforts. Provide a tracking sheet, such as that displayed in Exhibit 4.1, to your telephone operators and other staff members assigned to handle inbound patient calls and ask these "call trackers" to capture inbound call volume by day of week and time of day.

> **BEST PRACTICE**
>
> TRACK THE VOLUME OF REPEAT CALLS TO YOUR PRACTICE. A HIGH VOLUME OF REPEAT CALLS IS A SIGNAL THAT YOUR PRACTICE CAN IMPROVE TELEPHONE OPERATIONS AND PROVIDE MORE TIMELY PATIENT ACCESS. IDENTIFYING AND REDUCING REPEAT CALLS TRANSLATE INTO HIGHER PATIENT SATISFACTION AND LESS WORK FOR THE PRACTICE.

Be sure that your call trackers mark any calls that are repeat calls—that is, the caller has called once (or more) previously without getting resolution to his or her question. To do this, ask call trackers to make a special mark on the log whenever patients indicate that they have already called about the issue. If you are using automated system reports rather than a manual tracking log, you may want to supplement

[EXHIBIT 4.1] Inbound call volume—day of week and time of day

Hour	Monday	Tuesday	Wednesday	Thursday	Friday	TOTAL
8 a.m.–9 a.m.						
9 a.m.–10 a.m.						
10 a.m.–11 a.m.						
11 a.m.–12 p.m.						
12 p.m.–1 p.m.						
1 p.m.–2 p.m.						
2 p.m.–3 p.m.						
3 p.m.–4 p.m.						
4 p.m.–5 p.m.						
TOTAL						

[EXHIBIT 4.2] Inbound calls by day of week

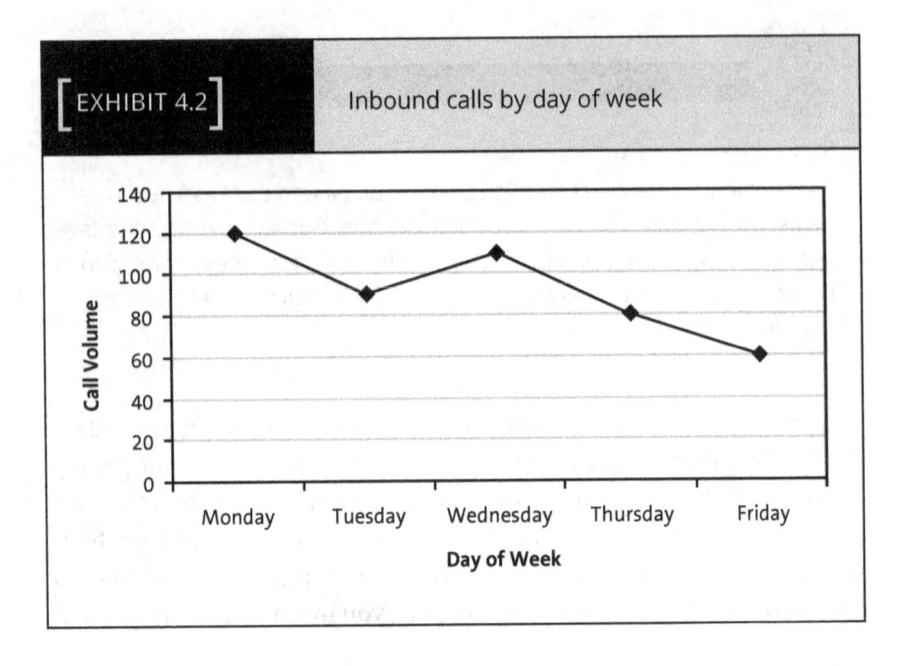

these reports with manual tracking of repeat call volume. By capturing data about repeat calls, you learn about changes that may be needed for more timely patient access. Repeat calls are not only frustrating for patients, but also represent unnecessary rework and staff inefficiencies.

When you have collected this information, graph the data by day of week, and look for trends. An example of a telephone graph based on inbound call volume by day of week is provided in Exhibit 4.2. As this example demonstrates, this medical practice receives a high call volume on Mondays and Wednesdays, tapering off through the rest of the week. This is a common pattern experienced by many medical practices.

Next, graph the data by time of day to identify trends. A sample graph of inbound telephone calls by time of day is reported in Exhibit 4.3. In this medical practice, we learn that call volume peaks at two times during the day—at 10 a.m. and also at 1 p.m. It is evident from the graph that the telephones are "closed" during the lunch period; as we discuss further in Chapter 5, transferring the callers to an answering service or routing them to voicemail at lunch or any other time of the

[EXHIBIT 4.3] Inbound calls by time of day

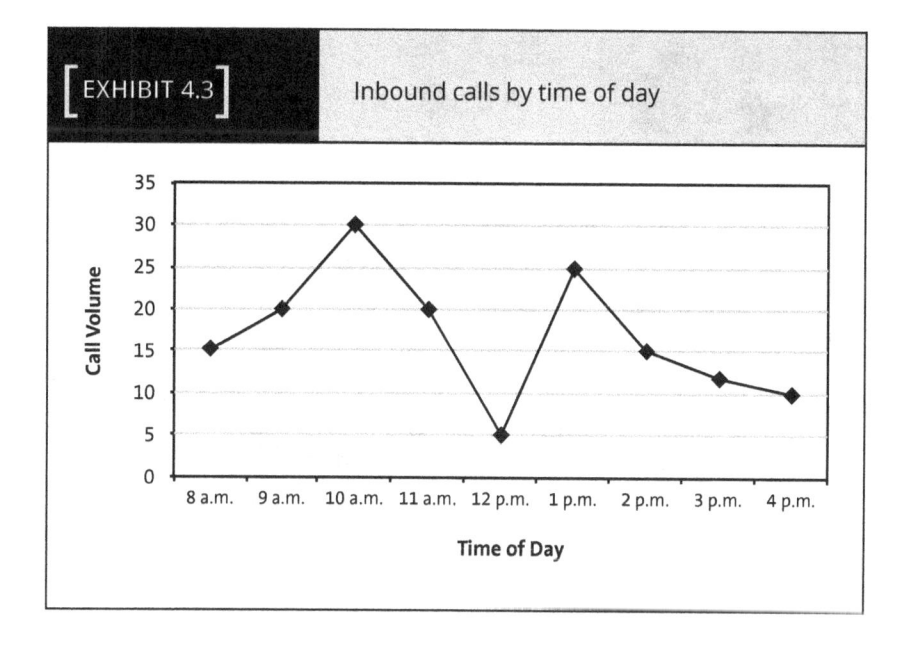

day simply batches and delays the work of telephone management in a medical practice.

The graph in Exhibit 4.4 adds the data captured for repeat call volume. You can easily see from the graph that patients are initiating repeat calls with high frequency at the end of the day. This is a signal that this medical practice is not meeting patients' expectations for call turnaround times. Patients are waiting throughout the day for a response to their calls and are initiating a second (or third) call to the practice by the day's end.

There may be many reasons for the uptick in repeat calls at the end of the day, but this trend most often indicates a problem related to the processing of work. Calls aren't being returned; patients are calling back to leave another message, to determine why their call isn't being returned, or to simply express their frustration at the lack of communication. The problem may stem from a provider who fails to take care of any messages during the day, instead batching the messages to address after office hours. It could also be a staffing issue, based on a medical assistant who is trying to room patients and support a physician

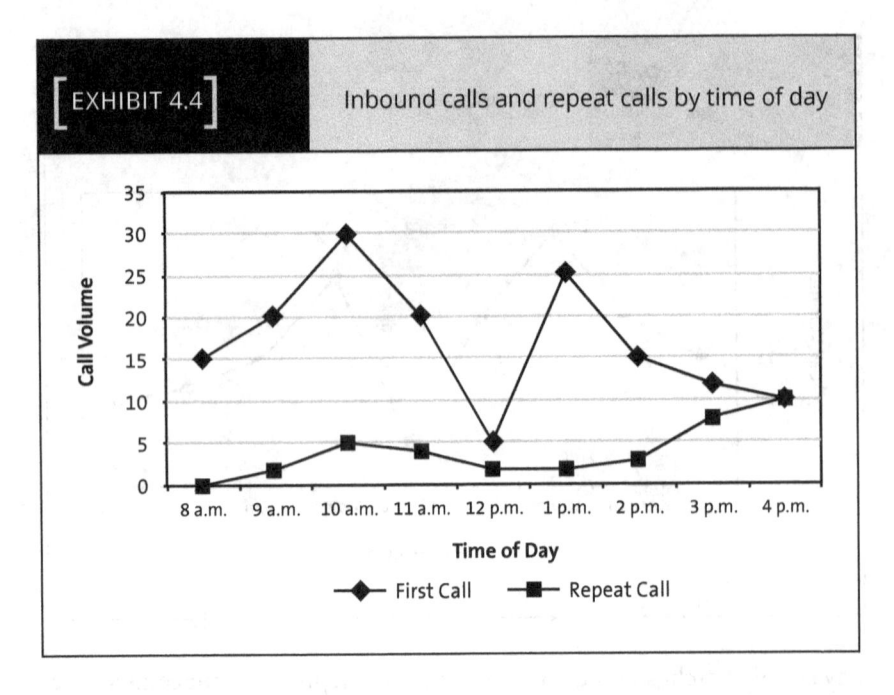

[EXHIBIT 4.4] Inbound calls and repeat calls by time of day

Time of Day	First Call	Repeat Call
8 a.m.	15	0
9 a.m.	20	2
10 a.m.	30	5
11 a.m.	20	4
12 p.m.	5	2
1 p.m.	26	2
2 p.m.	15	3
3 p.m.	12	8
4 p.m.	11	11

during a busy clinic session while being responsible for all inbound telephone calls. Whether the basis is work habits or simply not enough people to get the job done, the situation presents an opportunity for performance improvement. Identifying and reducing these repeat calls translates into higher patient satisfaction and less work for the practice.

Reasons for inbound calls

Now that you know your inbound call volume by day of week and time of day, the next step is to learn why patients are calling your medical practice. This provides the information you need to improve how you manage each type of call.

Although your telephone system may report your inbound call volume, it typically is not able to electronically report the reasons for inbound calls. If you have an automatic call distributor (ACD), you may be able to learn the volume of callers who pressed "1" for scheduling, "2" for the nurse, and so forth, but that does not give you the exact reason for the inbound call. For example, a call to the nurse could be a patient seeking test results or a patient who has a question about a medication. To capture the reasons for inbound calls, use a manual tracking form.

Ask all staff members who manage inbound telephone calls to keep a tracking form by day and time for a one-week period. Make sure that the week is generally representative of the call volume your practice experiences. Remind the call trackers each morning and several times throughout the day to keep monitoring the calls. Although you are not looking for statistical perfection, it's important not to underestimate the volume of inbound calls or miss an important category of calls.

To make the job easier, provide a form that allows call trackers to check off the most common reasons for inbound calls. A tracking form that details the reasons for inbound calls is provided in Exhibit 4.5 (if call tracking is available, establish 'reason codes' and use them to monitor calls).

It is also important to capture the calls managed by the clinical staff members who have telephone responsibilities. It may take some thought to capture an accurate count of inbound telephone data when you add the clinical staff as call trackers. Contemplate this scenario: your medical practice's telephone operators "screen" incoming calls and then transfer some of them to the clinical support staff, but established patients may also call the triage line directly. Consider the flow of work related to inbound calls to ensure that all calls are being captured, but that none are being double counted. Having the detail regarding the reason for the clinical call, however, is so important that it is worth your time to design a call tracking system that results in accurate data. You may also be able to retrospectively review and abstract the clinical messaging intake forms from your electronic health record (EHR) system to report the reasons for the calls.

After you have captured the reasons for your inbound calls, you have the data needed to manage your telephones, staff your telephones, convert inbound calls to outbound calls, and work to reduce telephone demand—all topics that we discuss in later chapters of this book.

EXHIBIT 4.5 Sample inbound call tracking form

Name: _____ Date: _____

Hour	Nurse/Physician	Billing	Referrals	Rx	Test Results	Personal	Appt.	Referring Physician	Other
8 a.m.–9 a.m.									
9 a.m.–10 a.m.									
10 a.m.–11 a.m.									
11 a.m.–12 p.m.									
12 p.m.–1 p.m.									
1 p.m.–2 p.m.									
2 p.m.–3 p.m.									
3 p.m.–4 p.m.									
4 p.m.–5 p.m.									

BEST PRACTICE

IF THE PERCENTAGES OF OUTBOUND CALLS BY TOPIC MATCH THOSE OF INBOUND CALLS, LOOK FOR A BETTER WAY TO MANAGE THAT TYPE OF CALL BY LEVERAGING TECHNOLOGY AND STREAMLINING COMMUNICATION.

Outbound Calls

Medical practices benefit by monitoring outbound telephone data. Develop a tracking process similar to that which is used for inbound telephone calls. Ask staff to record the volume of outbound calls, ideally by day of week and time of day. It's also helpful to understand the reasons for the calls. If the percentages of outbound calls by topic match up with those of inbound calls, there is likely some room for improvement in managing that particular type of call. For example, a high volume of inbound and outbound calls dealing with test results may indicate that your staff and patients are spending too much time playing telephone tag with each other trying to communicate test results. This finding signals that you should seek ways to leverage technology and streamline communication solutions for test results reporting, which we discuss in Chapter 5.

Additional call volume data

As part of data analysis regarding call volume, calculate two additional measures: (1) call volume by staff member and (2) the ratio of call volume to daily encounters. The call volume by staff member gives you insights regarding the work variability among your staff, which is useful when staffing the telephones (Chapter 6).

By calculating your ratio of inbound calls to encounters, you learn the magnitude of opportunity you may have to improve telephone management. The call volume to daily encounters ratio helps you to recognize the hassle factor associated with your telephones for patients and staff alike.

Although the volume of calls varies by practice, our research has shown that call volume is typically four to five times the number of patient visits per day. So, for example, if your practice sees 100 patients a day, then your call volume likely ranges from 400 to 500 calls per day.

We recommend an inbound telephone volume goal of only twice the number of patient visits, a goal achieved by practices that are successful at managing their telephones, reengineering their work processes, and deploying technology to enhance patient communication. To meet that goal, consider the following action:

- Focus on anticipating patients' needs so they do not have to resort to calling you.
- Contact patients before they call you. It's much more efficient for you to take charge of the process of communicating with patients, rather than waiting for them to communicate with you.
- Provide patients with other access channels to obtain information rather than relying on the telephone, such as secure communication through a patient portal.

We discuss these and other telephone improvement methods in subsequent chapters.

BEST PRACTICE

INBOUND CALL VOLUME IS TYPICALLY FOUR TO FIVE TIMES THE NUMBER OF PATIENT VISITS PER DAY...WHEREAS IT SHOULD BE APROXIMATELY TWICE THE NUMBER OF PATIENT VISITS—A GOAL ACHIEVED BY PRACTICES THAT ARE SUCCESSFUL AT MANAGING THEIR TELEPHONES, REENGINEERING THEIR WORK PROCESSES, AND DEPLOYING TECHNOLOGY TO ENHANCE PATIENT COMMUNICATION.

You may choose to evaluate additional information regarding call volume, but the measurements displayed in Exhibit 4.6 offer valuable insight into the challenges you face—and the opportunities available—related to your telephones.

Telephone Quality and Service Expectations

In addition to the volume of inbound telephone calls and the reason for the calls, you also need to examine the quality of your telephone management. Exhibit 4.7 summarizes key telephone quality measures. Much of these data are available electronically via your telephone system, such as the measures of abandonment rate, service level, and average speed to answer. Check with your telephone vendor for these options, using this list and the following definitions to guide your data-gathering efforts. Your telephone vendor may also have suggestions for other metrics, particularly for a large call center.

Key quality measurements and their definitions are provided here.

Abandonment rate. Abandonment rate is the percentage of total calls from patients and other callers that were disconnected by the caller prior to speaking with a telephone operator, either because they were not answered, the caller chose to disconnect, or the callers were placed on hold and then elected to disconnect the call. The abandonment rate is measured by comparing the portion of calls that abandon during a defined period of time compared with all calls received (to include those not answered) during that same time period. Practices typically measure both the number of abandoned calls as well as the percentage of calls that abandon. These data are available from a report generated from the telephone company, ACD, or the system's reporting software. The call abandonment rate is a typical measure of telephone performance, but it is not entirely under the telephone operator's control. Although abandoned calls are affected by the average wait time in the queue (which can be controlled by a telephone operator or call center), a multitude of other factors influence this measure, such as caller error in initial call placement, caller time tolerance, and availability of service alternatives.

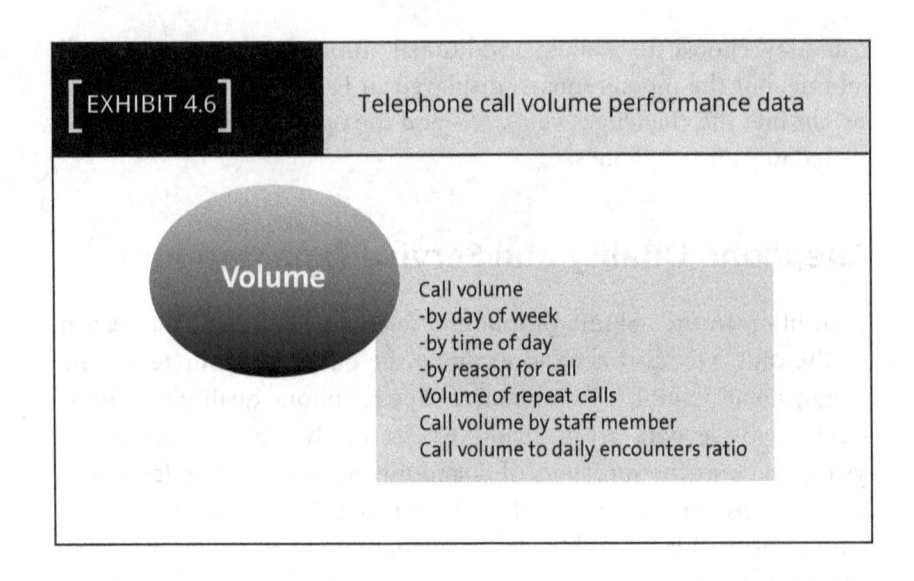

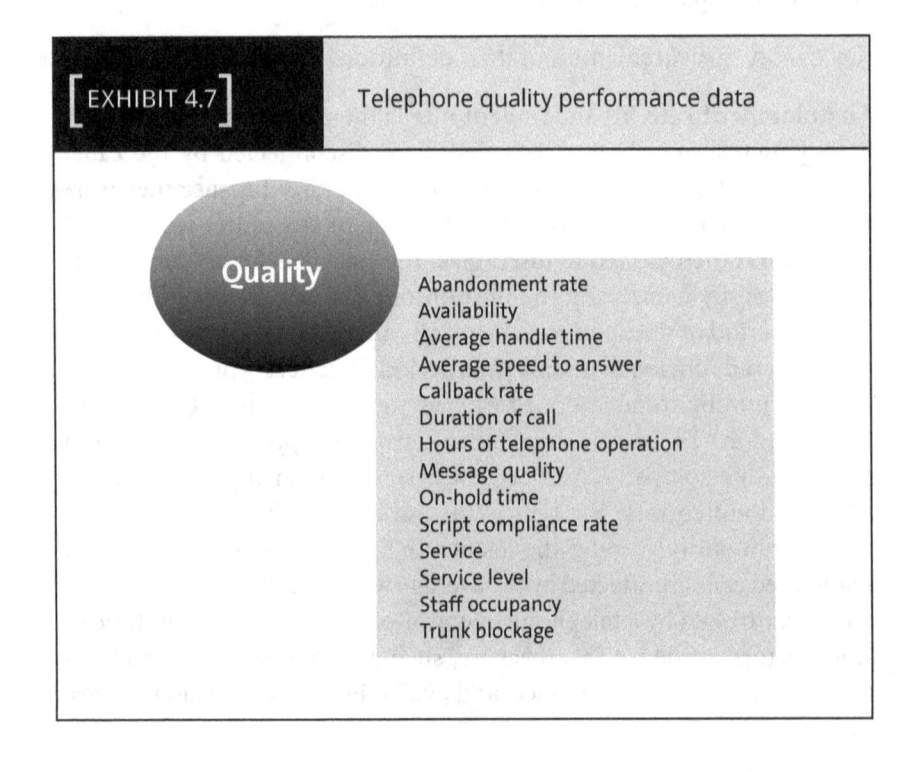

[EXHIBIT 4.6] Telephone call volume performance data

Volume
- Call volume
  - by day of week
  - by time of day
  - by reason for call
- Volume of repeat calls
- Call volume by staff member
- Call volume to daily encounters ratio

[EXHIBIT 4.7] Telephone quality performance data

Quality
- Abandonment rate
- Availability
- Average handle time
- Average speed to answer
- Callback rate
- Duration of call
- Hours of telephone operation
- Message quality
- On-hold time
- Script compliance rate
- Service
- Service level
- Staff occupancy
- Trunk blockage

We often witness an average abandonment rate of 10 percent among medical practices. We recommend a goal of 5 percent or lower.

Availability. Availability is the percentage of time that staff members are "logged in" to answer calls. The metric can be calculated by dividing the hours the staff members are logged onto the telephone system into total work hours. Availability, which is affected by the amount of time that a staff member is scheduled, as well as the time that he or she takes breaks and conducts other off-the-telephone activities, is an essential indicator to ensure that the expected staffing model is effective. Availability may be measured based on all staff, by site or team, or by individual employee. As we discuss in Chapter 7 on Call Centers, when accounting for standard breaks (including lunch), the most efficient state of a dedicated telephone operator is 85 percent productivity per workday.

Average handle time. The average handle time is the duration of the call plus after-call work. Available from the ACD, the average handle time should be measured and identified by time of day as well as day of week. Although handle times vary based on the type and content of the call, a staff member should typically deliver a consistent handle time within an acceptable range. Having a high average handle time, particularly when employees are all answering the same types of calls, can identify staff with performance improvement opportunities. For example, a telephone operator may take longer than his or her colleague if the operator first handwrites the message and then types the message after the caller has hung up in comparison to colleagues who are able to type the message in "real time." The ability to work in an efficient manner is essential for a telephone operator, and one with a high average handle time as compared to the duration of the call signals the need for intervention. Although there is no standard industry benchmark for average handle time, internally tracking and comparing this measure among your telephone staff give you insights into staff performance.

Average speed to answer. This measure is the amount of time (usually expressed in seconds) the practice takes on average to answer a telephone call. Because the arrival rate of calls can vary dramatically during the day, the average speed to answer is useful to assess and compare during multiple periods of the day that may have markedly different call volume amounts. Typically observed in half-hour increments, the average speed to answer is important to determine the variability of time required to answer the call. This measure helps you recognize the periods of the day where the average speed to answer is, for example, five seconds, and those periods in which the factor averages five minutes. Because the daily average as a whole may be reasonable, practices should observe the average speed to answer in half-hour increments to ensure that the needs of all callers are met throughout the day. If the average speed to answer is high, it's most common that other quality measures (for example, abandonment rate and service level) also reveal poor performance. These measures help to determine staffing changes that may need to be made to meet inbound call demand. Although there is no industry standard related to the speed to answer, we recommend that the average speed to answer the call not exceed 30 seconds, recognizing that the cycle of each ring is six seconds. Thus, the traditional phrase of "answer a call within three rings" could be translated into "answer a call within 18 seconds." Industry studies have revealed that callers typically abandon their calls after five to six rings, so the target you adopt for your medical practice should be at or below this level.

Callback rate. Two measures relate to the callback rate: first, the turnaround time for responses based on the time the messages or voicemails were left by callers (referred to as "callbacks") and second, the percentage of time that callbacks are being made based on the practice's protocols. Given the importance of callbacks from a clinical, risk management, and service perspective, the data regarding callbacks are important to measure. These callback rates are a function of multiple factors and a reflection of the quality of the external patient flow process for the practice as a whole. For example, the telephone operators must first take and distribute a quality message in a timely manner. Then the responder must act on that message in a timely manner. Callbacks are discussed in detail in Chapter 5. The industry standard is 30 minutes for clinical calls, and we recommend no more than three hours for all other calls. For nonclinical calls, the callback within the three-hour timeframe may be a response to confirm receipt of the message, with an answer provided to the caller by the end of the day.

Duration of call. Call duration is the amount of time that callers are on the telephone, measured either from the initial recording of the automated attendant or from when the call is taken by a live operator. This measure varies greatly based on the type of call. If duration becomes a significant factor of measurement for a medical practice, the result is that quality is often diminished as staff may be motivated to shorten calls. If callers believe that they are being rushed, they will not be satisfied. Moreover, an unintended consequence of placing too great an emphasis on call duration is that it may actually create more inbound call volume as patients call back to clarify their requests. Thus, we recommend that the duration of calls be tracked, particularly for staffing purposes, but this factor should not be used as a primary measurement of performance for telephone staff.

Hours of telephone operation. The hours of telephone operation are the normal hours your telephones are open and available to callers. Historically, the operating hours of the telephone have been limited to coincide with the practice's office hours (for example, 9:00 a.m. to 12:00 p.m. or 1:00 p.m. to 4:00 p.m.). However, today's medical practices are opening their telephones at least 30 minutes prior to the commencement of office hours and responding to their telephones through 5:00 p.m., including through the lunch period, with many of today's practices providing 24/7 access to nurse triage. To assess the effectiveness of your hours of telephone operation, measure the total number of inbound calls and the percentage of total calls that arrive outside of operating hours. To obtain information about calls arriving outside of normal operating hours, one can look at the number of voicemails left after hours, rely on hourly call reports generated by local and long-distance telephone providers, and/or review the call volume taken by your telephone answering service.

On-hold time. This measure reflects the amount of time a caller spends on hold during the course of the call. You can also observe the number of times a caller is placed on hold during the course of the conversation with the telephone operator. Like the other metrics, these on-hold data are available from your telephone system, ACD, or your reporting software. Obviously, the goal is to minimize the length of the on-hold time, as well as the number of times a caller is placed on hold. On-hold time is a function of several factors, but most notably the system's performance, staffing levels, and work processes. For example, a high percentage of on-hold time can indicate low staffing levels assigned to the telephone or insufficient knowledge by the telephone operators to respond to patient inquiries. There is no industry standard for on-hold time; however, we recommend that the on-hold time average 30 seconds or less. Many medical practices provide on-hold messaging—practice information or marketing "infomercials"—during the callers' on-hold time to occupy callers and assure them they are still in the calling queue.

Service level. The measure of service level is the percentage of calls that are answered within a pre-defined wait threshold, typically stated as X percent of calls answered in Y seconds or less. This factor can be reported as a simple, cumulative average over the day; a weighted average based on the actual calls per half-hour increment; or the percentage of half-hours in which the service level is met. This is perhaps the most widely used indicator of quality by call centers, yet there is no industry standard for service level. We recommend a minimum service level goal of 80 percent of calls answered within 30 seconds and a stretch goal of 80 percent of calls answered within 20 seconds.

Staff occupancy. Staff occupancy is the percentage of the logged-in time a staff member is actually busy on a call or performing after-call work. The metric can be calculated by dividing these "active" hours into total work hours. If staff occupancy is too low, staff members likely have idle time; if occupancy is too high, staff may be overworked. Staff occupancy tends to improve with the volume of the telephone operation. With a high volume of calls, there is a greater probability that there is another call to handle as soon as a telephone operator is finished with a call. As the volume of calls grows, increased economies of scale come into effect, translating into higher rates of staff occupancy. Although there is no industry standard, we recommend that staff occupancy exceed 80 percent. It is notable, however, that lower staff occupancy rates may be acceptable, particularly if the practice wishes to maintain a high level of quality. Of course, practices should be prepared to provide additional responsibilities for staff members, such as opening and processing mail, responding to online appointment requests, and so forth, during idle time. The volume of these extra tasks depends on the staff occupancy related to telephone work.

Trunk blockage. Trunk blockage is the percentage of callers who receive busy signals when trying to contact your medical practice. Trunk blockage data can be generated by the practice's ACD, or by its local or long-distance carriers. Although businesses tend to seek a goal of no more than 2 percent of inbound telephone calls blocked, it's not uncommon for practices to set a goal of having enough lines so that incoming calls are never blocked by busy signals. We recommend 0 percent trunk blockage for a medical practice.

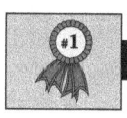

BEST PRACTICE

MAKE SURE YOUR CALLERS RECEIVE A CONSISTENT CALL-HANDLING EXPERIENCE. PATIENTS WILL PERCEIVE THE QUALITY OF YOUR MEDICAL PRACTICE BASED ON THEIR SERVICE EXPERIENCE WITH YOUR TELEPHONE STAFF.

We also recommend a number of other qualitative data regarding your telephones be routinely tracked and monitored. These include the following factors:

- **Service:** Compliance with expectations regarding high levels of professionalism, courtesy, compassion, and empathy; use of service recovery when applicable.
- **Script compliance rate:** Adherence to protocols regarding telephone scripts.
- **Message quality:** Compliance with protocols established by the practice regarding the accuracy, timeliness, grammar, and comprehensive nature of a message.

Ensuring that each caller receives a consistent call-handling experience regardless of the employee involved in the telephone communication is essential to a caller's perceived quality of his or her contact with your medical practice. Data regarding adherence to telephone procedures, call scripts, and message quality are not available from your telephone system reports. Instead, these factors are typically assessed through both general observation and a more formal quality-monitoring process (for example, mystery patient telephone surveys such as those discussed later in this chapter).

Recommended service standards for telephone-related patient access metrics are reported in Chapter 11 of this book: Key Performance Indicators. Use these as a starting point and develop your own service expectations related to your telephones. In some cases, you may need to determine interim goals, measuring progress to these goals before an "end-state" goal can be achieved. In most medical practices, steady and sure improvement over time is a goal that can be readily achieved.

It is important to recognize, however, that for some medical practices the telephones are so "broken" that dramatic improvement in a short period of time is needed to avoid losing patients through outmigration.

Customer Feedback

To enhance the quality data reported from your telephone system, we recommend the use of patient and referring physician surveys, mystery patient surveys, and patient advisory groups to help you understand the quality of your telephone management. Develop specific questions to request feedback from patients and referring physicians regarding your telephone operations and communication in general. Make sure your patient surveys include questions regarding telephone access and service. For example, include questions such as:

- "Is our staff courteous?"
- "Are they knowledgeable?"
- "Is the waiting time acceptable for calls to be answered?"

- "Can you generally get through on the telephones?"
- "Are you getting an appointment within the time frame you expected?"

These data give you information regarding how your telephone practices are perceived by your patients. These tools will help you move from anecdotal data regarding service quality to specific data allowing you to target areas for improved telephone quality.

> **BEST PRACTICE**
>
> THERE IS NO BETTER WAY TO OBTAIN PATIENT FEEDBACK THAN TO ASK YOUR PATIENTS DIRECTLY ABOUT THEIR EXPERIENCE WITH YOUR TELEPHONE STAFF. MAKE IT PART OF YOUR WORKDAY TO SIT DOWN WITH PATIENTS IN THE RECEPTION AREA AND ASK PROBING QUESTIONS ABOUT THEIR PERCEPTION OF YOUR PRACTICE.

Mystery patient telephone survey

In addition to conducting a patient satisfaction survey, implement a mystery patient telephone survey. Exhibit 4.8 provides an example of a mystery patient telephone survey. Use this as a starting point for your own survey. If you serve as the mystery patient, do not call from the practice's telephone, your home telephone, or any other telephone number that might be readily recognized by the practice's caller identification (ID) system.

Ask a friend or colleague to call your practice to learn how often he or she gets busy signals, how long he or she waits on hold, what he or she hears while on hold, and his or her impressions of the staff member answering the telephone. The staff members should not be told that the survey is being conducted so that their typical telephone practices can be evaluated.

If possible, have the surveyor attempt to call the practice during each hour block, that is, 7:00 to 8:00 a.m., 8:00 to 9:00 a.m., and so forth, throughout the day. You may be surprised—and not always pleasantly—by what happens when callers telephone during the lunch hour, immediately after the practice opens in the morning, or just before closing.

BEST PRACTICE

USE A MYSTERY PATIENT TELEPHONE SURVEY TO LEARN WHETHER TELEPHONE MANAGEMENT IS OPTIMIZED FOR YOUR PRACTICE.

Follow these steps to get the most out of your mystery patient survey.

- **Identify your goals.** Before you start, identify the key information you want to learn from the survey. For example: Is our staff courteous? Are they knowledgeable? What is the waiting time for calls to be answered? Must patients repeat their information or question(s) during the call?

- **Prepare the survey.** Use the "Mystery Patient Telephone Survey" (see Exhibit 4.8) as a starting point to develop your own mystery patient survey. Although having a mystery patient call your practice one time is a start, it's best to have a sample from which to draw. Conduct the mystery patient telephone surveys over a period of at least one month, with a minimum of 30 calls accomplished.

- **Find the mystery patient(s).** Depending on the purpose of your investigation, find a patient volunteer, ask a family member or colleague to help, or hire a consultant. Unless you're hiring experienced professionals, set clear expectations and ensure that they have a script to work from when they are

[EXHIBIT 4.8] Mystery patient telephone survey

Pick one of these sample questions:
- ☐ *Can you give me directions to your office?*
- ☐ *Can you tell me what experience Dr. _____ has?*
- ☐ *Do you accept _____ insurance?*
- ☐ *How long would I have to wait to get a physical exam with Dr. _____?*

Practice name: _____ Caller: _____

Call date: _____ Call time: _____

Overall impression:
☐ Exceeds standards ☐ Meets standards ☐ Does not meet standards

Was the telephone number easy to find on the practice's website?
☐ Yes ☐ No ☐ Not applicable

Number of rings: ☐ 1 ☐ 2 ☐ 3 ☐ 4 or More

Courtesy of the person answering telephone:
☐ Very pleasant ☐ Pleasant ☐ Rude or hurried

Did the person answering the telephone give you his or her name?
☐ Gave name clearly ☐ Gave name rapidly or mumbled ☐ Did not give name

Did the person answering the telephone give you the practice's name?
☐ Gave name clearly ☐ Gave name rapidly or mumbled ☐ Did not give name

Were you put on hold? ☐ Never put on hold
☐ Briefly put on hold after being asked if OK ☐ Put on hold without being asked

If you were put on hold, how long did you wait?
☐ Less than 30 seconds ☐ 30 to 90 seconds ☐ More than 90 seconds

If you were put on hold, did the staff member communicate with you about your estimated wait time? ☐ Yes ☐ No ☐ Not applicable

Level of knowledge of the person answering telephone:
  ☐ Extremely knowledgeable: gave complete, correct information immediately
  ☐ Knowledgeable: gave correct information
  ☐ Gave incorrect information

Was a message taken for someone to call you back?
  ☐ Message not taken: call handled by first person
  ☐ Message taken appropriately: received callback in specified time
  ☐ Message taken inappropriately: call not returned in specified time

(continues)

[EXHIBIT 4.8] Mystery patient telephone survey (continued)

Were you transferred to another individual who ultimately answered your question?
☐ Not transferred: call handled by first person
☐ Transferred once to correct person with appropriate explanation
☐ Transferred more than once, transferred to wrong person, or transferred without appropriate explanation

Courtesy of the person answering question:
☐ Very pleasant   ☐ Pleasant   ☐ Rude or hurried

Did the person answering the question give his or her name?
☐ Gave name clearly   ☐ Gave name rapidly or mumbled   ☐ Did not give name

Were you put on hold by the person who answered the question?
☐ Never put on hold
☐ Briefly put on hold after being asked if OK
☐ Put on hold without being asked

If you were put on hold by this person, how long did you wait?
☐ Less than 30 seconds   ☐ 30 to 90 seconds   ☐ More than 90 seconds

Knowledge of the person answering the question:
☐ Extremely knowledgeable: gave complete, correct information immediately
☐ Knowledgeable: gave correct information
☐ Gave incorrect information

Level of concern of the person answering the question:
☐ Demonstrated high level of genuine interest in caller
☐ Demonstrated interest in caller
☐ Demonstrated little or no interest in caller

Did the staff member ask if there was anything else he or she could help you with?
☐ Yes   ☐ No   ☐ Not applicable

Comments to support ratings exceeding or not meeting standards:
_____
_____
_____
_____
_____
_____
_____

placing the calls and when they are queried by your staff to provide follow-up information.

- **Use a non-identifiable telephone number.** Regardless of who serves as the "mystery patient," establish a telephone with a non-identifiable number for the surveyor to use. Otherwise, your staff may begin to realize that the same number is calling over and over again.

The mystery patient telephone survey will not give you all the answers you need to fully assess the quality of your telephones, but it will provide more credibility to anecdotal information you hear from patients.

Combine the results of the mystery survey with reports produced by your telephone system and with other observations you receive related to your telephones to give a clearer picture of the strengths and weaknesses of your current telephone processes. For example, if the mystery survey reports more than three rings before the call is picked up, evaluate telephone system reports regarding the average speed to answer in order to determine if there is congruity between the two data elements. As another example, if the mystery patient survey reports poor service by a particular staff member, evaluate the time that the staff member is spending on the telephone during a call to see if that signals a hurried approach with the patient.

Patient advisory group

In addition to survey tools, practices are seeking feedback from a representative cohort of patients. Identify a small but interested group of patients from your active population and ask them to meet at your practice once per quarter. This patient advisory group (PAG) can not only give you valuable feedback about your telephone service, but also about other general aspects of your practice.

A patient satisfaction survey typically gives you a "score" related to your telephones, such as a score of "4" on a Likert scale ranging from 1 to 5, but a PAG offers you real "stories" regarding your telephones to help you translate the data to usable information so you can take improvement action. Consider adding others to the PAG, such as a human resources director from a local employer; a practice manager from a referring physician; a parent, guardian, or family member of a patient with special needs; or another individual who is not a patient but may hear a lot of feedback about your practice. Prepare questions to ask. Listen carefully to the answers and comments, and take a lot of notes. In addition to providing invaluable feedback, a PAG signals to the community that you are trying to improve, which can make a positive impression. Particularly for telephone staff members who do not have face-to-face interactions with patients, consider inviting members of the PAG to come speak with staff members regarding their experiences with your practice. This "real-life" feedback makes a significant impression on staff.

BEST PRACTICE

DON'T ALWAYS RELY ON YOUR OWN IMPRESSIONS; LET THE VOICE OF THE CUSTOMER SPEAK LOUD AND CLEAR.

When asked to provide feedback, mystery patients—or your own patients and families—can be wonderful resources to your practice as you seek to improve telephone service, access, and operations. Don't always rely on your own impressions; let the voice of the customer speak loud and clear.

Now that you have measured the quality of your telephones, determine the expected service you want callers to receive when they contact your medical practice. Then measure the gap between your current state and your expectations. This gap analysis can guide you in your telephone redesign efforts.

BEST PRACTICE

What are your expectations for the telephones? Compare your current performance with your expectations and perform a gap analysis.

Summary

Measure your inbound call volume and the reasons for telephone calls to your practice. Analyze your current quality in comparison to your expectations. In this era of constrained resources, there will always be a challenge in managing the balance of volume and quality. With careful monitoring, you can achieve the balance that provides the level of service access that your patients and referring physicians expect. Armed with this data, it is possible to localize the source of telephone problems—be it system, staff, process, or service—and make access improvements. In the next chapter, we use the reasons for inbound telephone calls and share best practice tools to help you manage your telephones for improved results.

CHAPTER 5

Telephone Access Redesign

When you recognize the gap between your performance and expectations, you are in a position to take action to redesign your telephone processes for improved access. When call volume is beyond manageable levels or if patients can't easily access your practice and maneuver through the telephone system, practices have traditionally resorted to solving the problem by adding more telephone lines, buying new equipment, or hiring more staff. These steps may be necessary, but there are other options that need to be explored. Before adding to your practice's current telephone infrastructure, look for ways to improve call management and reduce telephone demand.

In this chapter, we discuss the key reasons for inbound telephone calls and present methods to:

- Better manage inbound calls based on reason for the call;
- Replace an inbound call with an outbound call; and
- Reduce inbound call demand.

This chapter's recommendations are intended to enrich communication with patients by eliminating the clutter and reducing delays in the channels of communication. By using our recommendations to better manage telephone demand, you can manage calls more efficiently and effectively. Furthermore, in some cases, you can turn the need for an inbound call (one that a patient or other caller initiates) into an outbound call (one that your practice initiates), and, in doing so, take control of your patient flow process. By focusing on changing telephone demand–for example, by reducing the need for patients to call—you may discover just how your practice unintentionally contributes to your current telephone problems with high call volume, long waits, and unhappy patients.

> **BEST PRACTICE**
>
> DON'T JUST ADD MORE STAFF OR UPGRADE YOUR TELEPHONE SYSTEM. REDESIGN YOUR PROCESSES TO IMPROVE TELEPHONE SERVICE, CONVERT AN INBOUND CALL TO AN OUTBOUND CALL, RESOLVE THE PATIENT'S NEEDS ON THE FIRST CALL, AND STRIVE TO REDUCE OVERALL INBOUND CALL DEMAND.

Engage Stakeholders

Distribute the results of your telephone analysis to physicians and staff. Engage them in discussions regarding the reasons for the performance. Although more staff can be hired to answer the telephone (and sometimes, that action is certainly necessary), the key is to focus on the processes that drive the calls. Conduct brainstorming sessions to explore actions to improve the management of telephone calls, as well as to determine methods to better anticipate the needs of patients and referring physicians and reduce telephone demand altogether.

> **BEST PRACTICE**
>
> ENGAGE STAFF AND PHYSICIANS IN REVIEWING TELEPHONE DATA AND DEVELOPING ACTION PLANS TO REDESIGN KEY WORK PROCESSES TO REDUCE TELEPHONE DEMAND.

Break down each category of inbound calls. Further analysis may show that a physician is telling patients to call back the following day to get their test results when, in fact, those results take more than 24 hours to be returned. Or you may discover that you need to do a better job of promoting the location of your new satellite clinic so that patients don't need to call for directions. Or, perhaps, you learn that you need to instruct patients to call their pharmacy, not the medical practice, for medication renewals.

Telephone Action Plan

Develop an action plan for telephone access redesign focused on telephone processes. Assign a staff member responsible for each action and develop an action time line. A sample action plan is provided in Exhibit 5.1. Initiate the plan in a stepwise fashion so that you don't overtax the action plan participants. Importantly, separately evaluate each phase of the plan. To ensure that you are on track for improvement, monitor call volume and quality both before and after implementing changes. If you do not see improvement, change tactics and try something else.

Telephone Management—by Call Type

We dedicate the rest of this chapter to review ideas for you to consider as you work to improve the telephone access to your practice. Let's now review key operational processes that drive telephone calls into a medical practice and explore best practices that can be used to better manage this call volume. In some instances, we present methods to replace an inbound call with an outbound call, thereby taking control of the communication process with the patient rather than assuming a more reactive approach. We also share how to reduce inbound call demand altogether by using other technologies and communication platforms with patients, referring physicians, and other callers.

Scheduling
To illustrate the connection between scheduling and poor telephone processes, let's review a common scenario. The receptionist transfers

[EXHIBIT 5.1] Sample telephone action plan

Goal	Action	Measure	Responsible Party	Time Line
Educate staff about telephone scripts.	Develop common scripts. Conduct educational program with telephone staff.	Mystery patient and patient satisfaction surveys regarding ease of telephone access.	Mary Smith	Weekly staff meetings in January–March. Measure outcome at first quarter surveys.
Reduce inbound calls for test results from 15% of inbound calls to 5% of inbound calls.	Provide patients with a take-home tool. Deploy automated test results reporting.	Number of inbound calls seeking test results.	Bob Jones – Tool. Cathy Johnson – Patient portal enhancement.	Within 30 days. Within 60 days.
Improve the response to the survey question "courtesy of telephone staff" from 90% satisfactory to 90% exceeds expectations.	Educate staff regarding customer service tools and techniques. Perform mystery patient surveys; provide feedback.	Patient survey results regarding telephone courtesy.	Harry Andrews – On-site education. Required reading: *Front Office Success* by Elizabeth Woodcock[1]	Within 30 days. Measure at next survey.
Reduce call abandonment rate from 7% to 3%.	Analyze data; assess call volume and quality metrics; evaluate staffing.	Telephone system reports.	Tom Smith	Within 90 days.

a patient's call to the scheduler. The scheduler cannot determine if the patient is sick enough to "deserve" one of the practice's precious few open slots for acute appointments. Unable to make a decision, the patient is then transferred to the nurse. After the patient is asked to repeat his or her request for the appointment, the nurse puts the patient on hold to consult with the physician, and, finally, the patient is transferred back to the scheduler. What's the accumulated time for all of these transfers? It can easily take up to 30 minutes.

What is the value to the patient? None. The patient just wanted an appointment to see you.

BEST PRACTICE

ASK THE PATIENT UP FRONT: "DO YOU WANT TO BE SEEN?" TURN NURSE TRIAGE CALLS INTO PATIENT VISITS (IN PERSON OR VIA VIRTUAL VISIT).

The healthcare delivery system in our country is in transition. On the one hand, most medical practices continue to receive fee-for-service reimbursement; thus, it is logical to turn telephone calls into encounters that can be billed. Some practices make it a rule to ask patients one of the following questions before the call is transferred to a nurse: "Do you want to be seen?", "Do you want to schedule an appointment?", or "Do you want to come in?" If patients are uncertain, the practice's staff can offer specifics regarding the availability, such as: "We have an appointment available with Dr. Jones this afternoon at 3 o'clock." That way, the practice is proactively turning un-reimbursable triage calls into reimbursable patient visits.

Accommodating patients on the schedule as they call with a desire to be seen is a scheduling method that is referred to as advanced access scheduling. This real-time access cuts down on the work associated with scheduling, as well as managing the burden that arises from deflecting patient demand. Without any triage involved, the patient is simply slotted in for an appointment the same day he or she requests to be seen.

On the other hand, as we transition our medical practices to new payment models to foster enhanced patient access beyond the face-to-face visit, the goal is to provide the best care at the right time in the most appropriate setting. Tying reimbursement to this goal leads us in the direction of providing care to some patients outside of the exam room, via telephone nurse triage; telehealth; and secure, electronic messaging with the care team. Changing the reimbursement system to emphasize prevention, outcomes, and quality will spark a revolution in telephone management, moving us from a generally passive approach—wait for the patient to call and then manage the call—to a proactive approach involving streamlined access and care outreach. Indeed, your practice can begin by deploying a nurse to act as a health coach or patient navigator for patients, or perhaps just taking the simple step of calling all of your patients who have been discharged from the hospital. Either way, you are positioning your telephones as a vital tool in the delivery and reimbursement systems of the future.

Scheduling templates

Beyond advanced access scheduling and prompting the patient to make an appointment, the scheduling template is often the cause of inefficient telephone processes. Many medical practices have worked hard to extend their scheduling templates 12 months into the future. This permits patients to be given a follow-up visit in one year. When patients exit the practice, they are provided with a written appointment card (or automated appointment slip) similar to that shown in Exhibit 5.2. But should we rely on a little card to ensure that the patient returns in 365 days? In this world of instantaneous access to information and automated calendar management, it is more than slightly problematic for practices to rely on a little card to ensure that a patient returns in a year.

For a significant number of these annual return visits, moreover, the patient's schedule or the physician's schedule will probably change in the ensuing 12 months—a likelihood that creates more work for

> [EXHIBIT 5.2] Annual appointment card

> **ACE MEDICAL**
> Dr. John Doe, Jr.
>
> _Kelli Weathers_
> has an appointment
>
> Date _Monday, Sept. 23_ at _8:45_ (AM) PM
>
> If you are unable to keep your appointment, kindly give us 48 hours notice, thank you.
> 555 Medical Way – Atlanta, Georgia 30033   404.555.1212

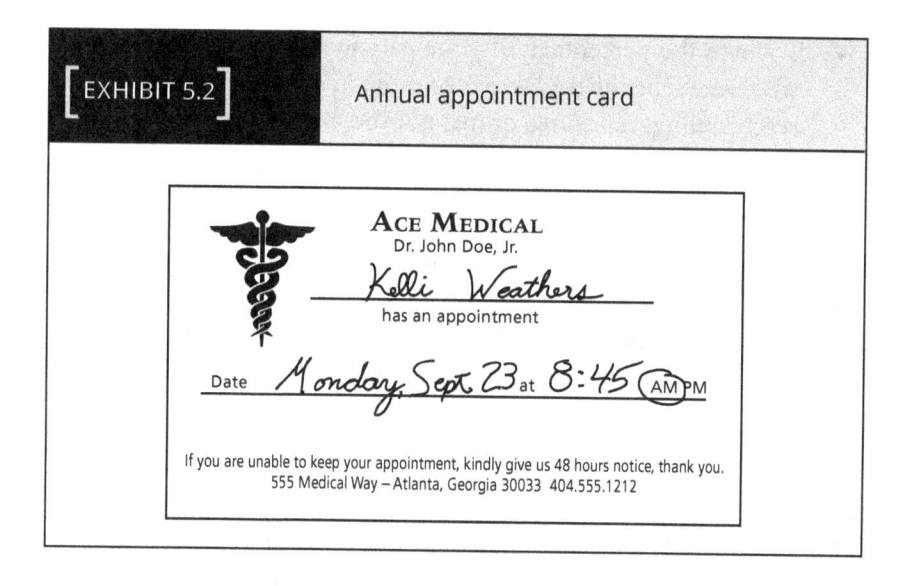

scheduling staff who then needs to bump and reschedule the patient, all the while playing telephone tag with the patient.

As we transition to reducing the hurdles associated with scheduling near-term appointments and accept the fact that we live in a world that demands immediacy—for example, same day or next day appointments—many medical practices are understanding their scheduling horizons - and limiting their scheduling templates to 12 weeks or less. In fact, some medical practices schedule only 30 days out. In this fashion, the telephone work associated with changes to the scheduling template is avoided. What also disappears is the blocked patient access caused when a slot—scheduled months earlier—appears to be full but will likely be cancelled by the patient (or perhaps, the physician). (See also Chapter 3: Scheduling Optimization for additional discussion of lag times to appointment.)

Gather the following data to determine the performance improvement opportunity related to scheduling in advance:

- Measure the success rate of your patients in keeping the appointments that were scheduled more than 12 weeks in advance;

- Evaluate the percentage of your patients with appointments who were scheduled 12 weeks or more in advance who end up rescheduling, canceling, or just not showing up; and
- Count those whom your practice bumps to another time slot because the provider's schedule changes.

If you determine that more than 50 percent of your patients fall into any of these categories, evaluate time periods other than 12 weeks in advance, such as appointments that are scheduled more than six weeks into the future. Again, determine if more than half of your patients fall into this new time category.

You now have the data to support changes to your scheduling horizon within your templates. We are not promoting turning away patients for their annual visit; instead, focus on appointment recall instead of scheduling. For example, determine a new template timeframe and establish an electronic recall list consistent with provider follow-up protocols. Place patients in your recall list 30 days before their requested appointments. So, if a patient seen in May 2018 needs to be scheduled for their next annual visit, inform the patient that he or she will be notified in April of 2019 via mail, electronic message, or telephone to call or go online to schedule their annual return appointment for May 2019. An outbound call to the patient—or a written or electronic notification—is easier and less costly than managing the chaos of the current scheduling—and rescheduling process. Further, self-scheduling reduces any requirements for staff involvement.

BEST PRACTICE

EVALUATE THE PERCENTAGE OF YOUR PATIENTS WHO END UP RESCHEDULING, CANCELING, OR NOT SHOWING UP. CONSIDER CHANGING YOUR SCHEDULING TEMPLATE TIME LINE IF THE PERCENTAGE IS GREATER THAN 50 PERCENT.

Self-scheduling

Another way to streamline scheduling—and reduce scheduling calls—is to permit patients to schedule appointments via your patient portal, chat, secure messaging, cellular-phone-based application ("app"), or a dedicated self-scheduling system. Regardless of the communication channel, three methods are adopted by medical practices that engage in "self-scheduling."

- **Appointment Request.** Self-scheduling involves a patient submitting an electronic message, text, chat, or other electronic message to your practice requesting an appointment (perhaps a general request or one for a specific date and time). After receiving the request, a staff member calls the patient to schedule the date and time or the practice responds to the patient in the same method that the patient initiated the request (electronic message, text, chat, or other technology). For example, if the patient sends a text message to the practice, the practice sends an electronic confirmation of the appointment to the patient via text or, if necessary, offers other date and time options to the patient.

- **Direct, Established-Patient Scheduling.** The patient is able to select a date and time and then slot themselves directly on the calendar (the schedule is blinded with regard to other patient names). This functionality is typically offered by the practice management system.

- **Open, New-Patient Scheduling.** The patient is able to determine the availability of a new patient appointment slot, and schedule into it. This functionality may be offered by the practice management system, or a third party vendor via a "bolt-on" to your system.

For both direct and open scheduling, the patient is in essence functioning as a virtual scheduler by directly scheduling an appointment in your system.

These self-scheduling offerings reduce inbound scheduling calls to your practice. Importantly, patients are able to schedule appointments with you at their convenience, even if it is after hours. Further, self-scheduling demonstrates a positive impact on no-shows. Given the engagement in scheduling the appointment date and time, the patient is more likely to show. Developing communication channels for patients that reduce reliance on the telephone to schedule appointments is a win-win for everyone.

Appointment reminders

Many medical practices have leveraged technology, through the use of vendor support, to remind patients of their appointment via an automated outbound call placed to the patient's preferred telephone number. More recently, this technology is being replaced by text messages to the patient's cellular phone or messages via the patient portal. Patients may also be requested to confirm via text message that they will keep their appointment. Leveraging technology tools to assist in the appointment reminder process reduces the need for staff to place outbound calls—and may lead to lower missed appointment rates for your practice.

Test results

Do your patients have the information they need to know when and how to expect their test results? In many cases, we have found that practices leave patients to guesswork, thus unintentionally encouraging a telephone call. For example, we observed a physician discussing several diagnostic tests she was about to order for her patient. When the patient asked when the results would be available, the physician said, "immediately." With this message in mind, the patient will likely place a call as soon as he completes the tests, perhaps even before they've been interpreted. It's also likely that the patient will continue to call—two or three times a day—until he gets the results or someone intervenes with a more accurate date and time.

Replace this scenario with the following general guidelines that best serve the patient:

- **Be realistic about test results.** Establish patients' expectations before they leave the exam room, and give yourself some wiggle room. If it's usually a 72-hour turnaround time to get a CT interpretation, for example, indicate that you'll communicate with the patient in four days. If the result of the test is abnormal, your practice will likely learn of it before the fourth day and, in turn, contact the patient in a manner and time dictated by the clinical circumstances. In this example, for both normal and abnormal results, you exceed the expectations of your patients if you call earlier than the fourth day. If you call later, however, it is likely that the patient will have already left you a message.

- **Institute formal tools.** Use resources to help patients understand when and how they will receive their test results. Use an EHR system's after-visit summary, the patient portal, or a test-specific card outlining the location of the test (including a map) and the approximate timing and communication of test results. Give information to the patient as a take-home tool, and then verbally confirm the information to the patient. This proactive approach helps the patient—and likely avoids an inbound call to your practice. Be sure to also provide written instructions to the patient regarding the test. A patient who is well informed about an upcoming test doesn't need to call back about directions to the facility or preparatory instructions. Your communication about the test can have a positive—or negative—impact on your telephone process.

- **Follow a standard test-reporting process.** It's simply unacceptable to tell a patient when ordering a test: "If you don't hear from us, everything is just fine." This protocol only generates myriad telephone calls or, even worse, a base of uninformed patients or a problem result that slips through the cracks and is not communicated to the patient. Use one of three notification methods to keep patients informed.

- **Mail results to patients.** Notify patients as to when to expect their results via the mail. Develop a standard notification letter, or mail a copy of the actual test results to the patient with a written note from the physician regarding interpretation and any further instructions or follow-up.
- **Obtain voicemail results permission.** For normal test results, obtain permission from the patient to leave a message on his or her voicemail. Exhibit 5.3 offers a sample permission statement.
- **Establish electronic test results reporting.** Instead of relying on a letter or voicemail message to disseminate test results, provide patients with secure access to their test results via a patient portal. The value of the portal is that the patient has a written account of the results that can be printed and/or shared with others. Importantly, a portal can display results from the same type of test, trended over time. For example, a patient's cholesterol level trended over time makes a more powerful impact than a data point in time. The patient can see in a visual form whether his or her health measures are improving or regressing and become more engaged in his or her health and wellness. Of course, you must continue to see patients in the office or place a call to those patients with abnormal results or findings that may impact current medications, physical restrictions, and other clinical issues, as medically appropriate. The notification of test results is also the best manner of obtaining interest and utilization of your patient portal.

The key is to control the process. While not all patients follow the instructions regarding these tools, even a reduction of 10 percent of the calls from patients trying to track down their results is a significant improvement in reducing the volume of inbound calls.

[EXHIBIT 5.3] Sample voicemail permission statement

I authorize PRACTICE NAME, its physicians and employees to leave detailed messages specific to my medical care, including test results, on the telephone number(s) listed below. I understand that when a voicemail message exists, it is no longer covered under the Health Insurance Portability and Accountability Act of 1996 and therefore is not protected from unauthorized access. This authorization is effective _____. I understand that this authorization can be revoked at any time by submitting a written request to PRACTICE NAME. Unless revoked sooner, this authorization to release detailed medical information will expire one (1) year from the effective date listed above. This authorization pertains to voicemail messages only and does not extend to family members and/or other persons that may answer the telephone. This authorization is not required to receive care at PRACTICE NAME. Patients opting not to sign this authorization will receive medical information such as test results personally rather than via a voice messaging system.

Telephone number(s): _____   _____

Patient signature:_____ Date: _____

(This is only a sample. Please consult with an attorney in developing a voicemail permission statement for your practice.)

When realistic expectations are set with the patient—particularly if the alternative is better communication of important information, such as the display of results via a portal—the patient is far less likely to place a telephone call to your practice. By setting realistic expectations with your patients, you then control the communication rather than react episodically throughout the day to inbound call demand.

BEST PRACTICE

YOU CAN SENSE SOMEONE'S ATTITUDE THROUGH THE TELEPHONE. MAKE A POINT OF SMILING AS YOU SPEAK—PATIENTS SENSE THAT SMILE—EVEN OVER THE TELEPHONE.

Prescriptions

Telephone calls regarding prescriptions and medications can overwhelm a practice. Not only are they significant in volume, but the workflow associated with a prescription-related call is also significantly encumbered for many practices. For example, we overheard a triage nurse listening to the prescription renewal line where one of their elderly patients—Ms. Mary Smith—had left a voicemail with the message that she wanted more of her 'little orange pills' called in to 'her' Walgreens. This initiated a time-consuming process: The nurse had to determine who the patient actually was, the medication that the 'little orange pills' represented, the appropriate dosage, and to which of the 23 Walgreens in their city the patient was referring. After that information was retrieved and the physician was consulted, then began the round of telephone tag as the nurse tried to reach the patient.

To reduce inbound calls—and improve the quality of prescription management—consider the following actions:

- **Determine the patient's preferred pharmacy**. Don't wait until the patient calls for a prescription renewal. Along with the patient's name, address, telephone number, and so forth, capture the patient's preferred pharmacy as a basic, essential data element that is always requested and documented at registration. Of course, just as demographic information may change, alterations to the preferred pharmacy should be documented if the patient requests a different pharmacy during a subsequent visit.

- **Leverage the pharmacy**. Replace the automated prescription line with direct patient-to-pharmacy communication. If you have historically accepted prescription calls over the telephone via a dedicated line, voicemail, or staff member, establish a new policy in writing that directs patients to their pharmacy instead of the practice. On your automated prescription line, place a message that explains the new process and assures patients that calling the pharmacy results in timely, accurate prescription management. Furthermore, include a timeline advising patients when to expect the completion of their renewal requests. If the pharmacy is sending text reminders to patients or otherwise communicating with patients when their prescription is ready, notify your patients regarding the pharmacy's communication process.

- **Develop an electronic interface with the pharmacy to "e-prescribe."** Request the pharmacists to securely, electronically transmit or fax the request for renewals to your medical practice. The advantages of electronic communication are that neither party has to wait on hold, and both parties have documentation for the patient's record.

- **Create an automated prescription renewal process.** Permit patients to request a prescription renewal via your patient portal, with the prescription then processed by your practice and electronically submitted to the pharmacy. The pharmacy then notifies the patient when the prescription is available.

- **Educate staff to differentiate between calls for prescription renewal and medication questions.** We often see messages taken for nursing staff or physicians that state "patient has questions regarding medication" when the patient is only seeking a prescription renewal. Of course, patients should be appropriately routed to the physician or nurse if they have a question about the medication itself; however, telephone staff should be asking sufficient information to learn the difference between these types of calls.

- **Evaluate your prescription writing protocols.** Call volume for prescription renewals varies by specialty and may fluctuate by time of year and day of week. Some practices, such as residency clinics, which typically write prescriptions for a shorter cycle, may have a much higher volume of telephone calls because patients run out of medications more quickly. If patients don't have a subsequent appointment, the only method of continuing their medication is to call and request a renewal. This process may impact the ability of some patients to take their prescribed medications, as they either forget or elect not to call when they run out. Of course, the standard of care and the needs of your patients should guide telephone operations, but it's an opportune time to evaluate your prescription writing protocols, particularly for maintenance medications. Consider holding a discussion regarding prescriptions, determining whether standard guidelines regarding prescriptions can be established, taking into account a patient's convenience and compliance, as well as the practice's prescription management process.

- **Ask patients to bring their medications to their appointments.** Asking patients to bring in their medications to their appointments helps clinical staff to accurately document the patient's medications, dosages, and termination dates. When patients bring their prescription bottles to the visit, it may add a few minutes to the visit; however, it saves time in the long run. Alternatively, ask the patient to write down their prescriptions (including dosages) and their termination dates and bring this with them to their appointments. A telephone call requesting a prescription renewal is more costly than managing the issue in "real time" at the time of the patient's appointment. Documenting the time and effort that physicians spend in managing the medications—a key driver in choosing the level of the evaluation and management (E/M) code you bill—may be an opportunity for additional revenue. If you adhere to documentation and coding guidelines, these efforts may not only benefit the patient, but also your practice's bottom line.

- **Flag pending renewals during visit preparation.** Steps can also be taken during the clinical preparation for the visit to identify prescriptions that may need to be renewed. The patient's medical record should be reviewed and any pending renewals flagged when the chart is prepared, which typically occurs one to two days prior to the encounter. Ideally, you would automate this process through your EHR.

- **Ask patients about medications during visits.** The easiest way to prevent inbound calls for prescription renewals is to perform a medication reconciliation at the time of the rooming or intake process of the visit. This helps ensure that the information is gathered and ready for the physician when he or she enters the exam room, and it integrates this work into your patient flow process. Many practices also set the stage for several opportunities to proactively ask patients about their renewals using a multifaceted approach: clinical staff during the patient intake and rooming process, the physician when he or she begins the encounter, and a staff member at check-out. However, rather than verbally prompting the patient multiple times during the visit, an EHR system permits each of the physicians and staff who interact with the patient to confirm that the prescription renewal has been addressed.

BEST PRACTICE

GIVE PATIENTS A PORTABLE TABLET IN THE RECEPTION AREA FOR THEM TO DOCUMENT QUESTIONS FOR THE PHYSICIAN AND IDENTIFY THEIR CURRENT MEDICATIONS.

- **Use reminder tools.** A significant number of renewal calls are from patients who have been seen in the last week—they simply forgot to ask you about their renewals while they were in the office, and importantly, your practice did not elicit this information. While patients wait in the reception area, hand them a clipboard or an iPad with a "Questions to Ask My Doctor" and "Medications That I Need to Discuss With My Doctor Today" form to complete. Another way to jog memories is to place a sign in each exam room asking about medications. As noted previously, collecting information about current medications from patients should be incorporated as an expected component of the rooming process.

- **Stage follow-up appointments based on medication renewals.** Time the patient's follow-up appointment within the prescription renewal period. For example, let's assume the physician prescribes 30 days worth of medications and asks the patient to come back in a month for a medication check. If there are no appointments available within 30 days (or the time period ends on a weekend), the patient might be scheduled to return outside of the 30-day window. If the patient is scheduled on the 33rd day, for example, the patient must call the medical practice to ask for a renewal for the three-day lapse. The result is extra work for staff and inconvenience for the patient. Even worse, it may also mean that patients go without necessary medication, potentially negatively impacting their care.

- **Use EHR system alerts.** Develop alerts, which are typically a function of clinical decision support tools, in the EHR system to remind the practice when the patient's medications are about to run out. This way, the practice controls the communication. For example, alerted by the EHR system, a staff member can communicate with the patient, stating: "Ms. Smith, Dr. Jones would like to see you in the next 30 days; we want to see how you are doing and review your medications." Being proactive avoids the situation where patients are able to obtain telephone-based prescription renewals for prolonged periods of time without being seen by the physician, and arguably results in better care.

- **Integrate the formulary.** Some prescription telephone calls may come from patients who discover that the medication prescribed was not on their insurance company's formulary. Prompted by sticker shock, they call back to seek an alternative medication. Practices with the ability to check the current formulary for each major insurance company with which they participate have decreased inbound telephone calls, streamlined patient flow by reducing interruptions to the physician, and reduced patient frustration.

- **Interface with a prescription monitoring program.** For the safety of patients, states are making available information regarding dispensed controlled substances by patient. These programs are assisting in the identification of patients who may be misusing or diverting prescription drugs, or those who may be at risk for detrimental interactions or overdose. Manual query of these databases may be required or requested by your state. Automate the process by integrating the workflow related to the prescription monitoring program into your EHR system and/or e-prescribing process. This provides for compliance with your state (if applicable), and avoids inbound telephone calls from the pharmacy, state, or other stakeholders in the event of a problem with an abusive patient.

- **Turn an inbound call to an outbound call.** Place follow-up calls to newly prescribed patients. Use an electronic tickler system to remind clinical staff to call patients soon after their visits if you suspect there could be any concern about the dosage, delivery, side effects, or efficacy of the medication you've just prescribed. Reinforce the habit of making these follow-up contacts with newly prescribed patients by discussing with your clinical team the most common questions you tend to receive.

The advantages of taking charge of the work related to medications stem far beyond reducing the number of inbound telephone calls. Performing the work at the time of the encounter is, of course, best for the patient and can lead to reduced errors related to managing the patient's medications and renewal processes. It is also best for your practice's bottom line, as the physician may be able to code for the work related to the medication by incorporating it into the level of the E/M visit. Performing the work during the encounter, instead of later in the course of a series of telephone calls, may result in a higher E/M level for the visit.

Patients can readily perceive dysfunction in a medical practice, and it can play a large role in patient assessment of your telephone service. For example, if a telephone operator handles repeat calls from a patient throughout the day and informs the patient that it is the clinical staff's fault for not promptly returning his or her calls, telephone operators are sharing the internal dysfunction of a medical practice. The importance of teamwork should not be overlooked. The level of patient satisfaction typically mirrors the level of staff satisfaction. Make sure your medical practice is functioning as a true care team.

Clinical advice and triage

Patients call the practice to receive clinical advice and triage. Before you add another triage nurse to manage these clinical calls, conduct a detailed review of the reason for medical advice calls. The inbound call data that we obtained in Chapter 4: Call Demand and Performance provide useful information regarding the reasons for inbound calls. One of the call categories in the tool presented in Chapter 4 is a global category titled "nurse/physician." To capture the questions patients pose related to clinical advice and triage, ask clinical staff to maintain a clinical calls log. A Clinical Calls Log and Instruction Guide are provided in Exhibit 5.4.

Use the Clinical Calls Log to evaluate where calls could be avoided altogether by improving patient education while patients are in the office. Further, scrutinize the calls regarding issues that may have been better handled in the office, face-to-face with a provider. You may be able to develop strategies to avoid many of those types of calls and conserve the staff time spent handling them. As patients seek more "telemedicine" and only a handful of insurance companies reimburse for it, your practice is stuck with the overhead related to handling those calls. If patients want or need to be seen, schedule them to be seen.

Physicians can help this process along. A physician's verbal assurance to the patient that his or her clinical associate, or the practice's health coach or patient navigator, is an important member of your team helps patients feel comfortable communicating with a team member. This

[EXHIBIT 5.4] Clinical call logs and instruction guide

Patient Name	Date of Call	Date of Last Appointment	Reason for Call
Mary Smith	07/16/19	07/13/19	What medications can she take on the day of her surgery?
Tom Green	07/16/19	07/12/19	His incision site is bleeding and he is not sure what to do.

To use the Clinical Call Log, follow these steps for best results:

1. Ask everyone in your practice who handles clinical calls to use the incoming clinical call log.
2. Record in the log the general purpose of each patient's call, the date of the call, and the date of his or her last appointment.
3. Keep the logs for a few weeks, then review the entries in the "Reason for Call" column. Group the frequently asked questions into basic categories. For example, a surgical practice may be able to group patient questions into:
   - Preoperative instructions: "Can I take my hypertension medication the day before surgery?"
   - Postoperative wound care: "What do I do if it's been three days since the surgery and the site is still tender?"
   - Logistics: "What time should I be at the hospital?"
   - General questions: "Can I drink alcohol with this medication?"
4. Count the patient questions in each category.
5. Note the time elapsed since the patient's last office appointment and highlight the calls received within one week of the patient's most recent office encounter.
6. Review the results with the physicians and support staff. Look for patterns. Note which categories have the most questions and which questions are asked most often.
7. Discuss how your practice can proactively educate your patients about the frequently cited categories, and pay particular attention to the questions asked by patients who were just seen in the office.
8. Perform the call logging exercise bi-annually and look for other trends.
9. Seek solutions to reduce call volume—and improve patient care.

also reduces the volume of telephone calls by patients who state: "I only want to talk with my doctor." A team approach to patient care and to managing inbound calls is becoming the norm.

> **BEST PRACTICE**
>
> THE BETTER EDUCATED YOUR PATIENTS ARE, THE MORE EFFICIENT YOUR MEDICAL PRACTICE CAN OPERATE.

The following strategies will help you implement tools to reduce clinical calls, as well as increase patient awareness.

- **Plan for the visit.** Establish a protocol for planned care visits: work to anticipate patients' needs by reviewing their records before they present. Identify their needs for recommended preventive care, including that which may have been missed at previous visits or simply based on the timing of the patient's last visit. After they present, proactively provide written information and resources to patients regarding their diagnosis, care, and treatment plan. Providing this support may be incorporated into the role of the nurse or medical assistant; it may also be the responsibility of a dedicated health coach or patient navigator. As clinical staff members become more involved in patient education, patients gain more knowledge about their care. Better educated patients are not just medically compliant, they help your practice to operate more efficiently and enhance your providers' ability to deliver quality medical care.

> **BEST PRACTICE**
>
> IMPLEMENT "PLANNED CARE VISITS"—PROACTIVELY REVIEW PATIENTS' RECORDS BEFORE THEY PRESENT. FOR PATIENTS RETURNING FOR A FOLLOW-UP VISIT, EVALUATE EXPECTED DOCUMENTATION FOR IMAGING, LAB, AND CONSULTANT

VISITS TO WHICH THE PATIENT WAS REFERRED AT THE PRIOR VISIT. ANTICIPATE PATIENTS' NEEDS BY DETERMINING AND OUTLINING RECOMMENDED CARE TO ADDRESS WITH THE PATIENT DURING THE VISIT.

- **Give patients a take-home tool.** Provide patients with a record of their visit, commonly known as an "after-visit summary." These documents can be provided in electronic or paper format to permit a patient to refer to his or her treatment plan.
- **Use e-communications.** Direct patients to your web portal for test preparations, preoperative and postoperative instructions, and other routine information.
- **Encourage questions.** Ask patients during or at the end of the appointment if they have questions about the visit. Consider introducing a health coach or patient navigator, upon the physician's departure from the exam room, to spend time with the patient regarding questions he or she may have.
- **Distribute handouts.** Offer patients a handout with websites, support groups, or other resources that you recommend. Direct them to web-based patient resources.
- **Inform your patients.** Proactively address the side effects of medications, procedures, or treatments with patients.
- **Develop individualized action plans.** Develop a plan (based on templates, where appropriate) for each patient regarding his or her treatment and present it to the patient in a notebook that includes a log for the patient to record details about his or her care. In lieu of a physical notebook, consider making the information available to the patient in electronic format via a patient portal or personal health record.
- **Develop a question-and-answer (Q&A) document.** Create a written Q&A form for the top five to ten questions patients have regarding a particular diagnosis, treatment, or procedure. Place the answers to frequently asked questions regarding the diagnoses or services provided most frequently to your patients on your practice's website or patient portal, or in a handout to distribute to patients.

- **Promote video resources.** Develop videos to discuss particular diagnoses, treatments, or procedures to supplement face-to-face conversations and written materials. The video can be professionally produced; however, making it more personalized to you and your practice has its benefits too. Create a video of yourself discussing an issue, such as post-operative wound care, and duplicate the video in a format that is current (AVI, F4V, WMV, etc.). Post the video on your website or social media and direct your patients to the link. The video can also be linked on your practice's website. Determine the best option for your practice, and, in addition, provide resources outside of the practice, such as support groups and websites.
- **Institute remote monitoring.** Send the patient home with a personal monitoring device, with instructions regarding connectivity and reporting results.

You can't—and don't want to—eliminate all of the clinical calls, but you can reduce the number of calls with a little effort.

BEST PRACTICE

VIDEOTAPE YOURSELF COMMUNICATING INSTRUCTIONS TO A PATIENT, AND POST IT ON YOUR WEBSITE OR SOCIAL MEDIA.

Frequent callers

Some patients have above-average needs for communicating with the practice. These patients—often referred to as "frequent callers" based on the repeated calls they make to the practice—may have chronic or complex illnesses, or perhaps their communication is based on an emotional need. Indeed, many practices assessing their clinical calls conclude that 80 percent of the work is driven by 20 percent of the patients. Instead of being frustrated by frequent callers or abandoning their needs, consider alternative strategies to meet their needs—and yours.

Identify frequent callers, and create and promote an alternative form of communication with the practice rather than resorting to the telephone. Alternative forms of communication include secure, encrypted electronic message, texting, or faxing an electronic form via a fax server. Some practices have determined that identifying these patients and proactively communicating with them has reduced inbound communication.

For example, if your physicians round at an assisted living facility, your practice may receive dozens of calls each week from the facility's staff communicating minor issues that are not emergencies but which must be reported. Instead, ask the facility to securely electronically message or fax the nonemergency injury reports to you. Better yet, give your physicians and other clinicians a means to access your EHR system from the facility so they can instantly review, handle, and document the reports while they're at the assisted living facility (or at other practice locations, such as satellite offices). If you maintain patients' records on paper, store those records at the facility and assign a physician to review, handle, and document the calls at the facility. Either method eliminates the administrative demands on staff members to manage a high volume of inbound calls, message-taking, and follow-up.

Frequent callers may not be particular patients, but rather driven by specific circumstances. For examples, patients who have been discharged by the hospital and/or just returned home from a procedure may exhibit a higher-than-average call rate. Instead of waiting for patients to call, initiate an outbound communication to those patients. Establish a process to ensure that the practice is notified on a daily basis of all patients discharged from the hospital (and perhaps other patients, such as those who presented to the emergency department), with outbound calls (or another effective form of communication) placed to each patient. This responsibility may be the function of the telephone nurse(s), health coach or patient navigator.

High-risk and chronic care patients

Patients with high-risk or chronic medical conditions who need ongoing care typically generate a high call volume. This patient population also tends to represent a significant number of hospitalizations, emergency department visits, and readmissions. In the new era of healthcare delivery, the practice is reimbursed based on reducing unnecessary visits at these high-cost facilities. To decrease this inbound call volume—and, more importantly, work to cut unnecessary hospitalizations, emergency department visits, and readmissions—consider the following actions:

- Provide proactive care coordination and outreach to patients by health coaches and patient navigators.
- Implement planned care visits to ensure that all information about patients is being received, documented, and reviewed, as well as the identification and facilitation of all recommended care.
- Provide tools and resources to assist patients, as well as their family members and caregivers, in self-management.
- Encourage patients to communicate via the patient portal, particularly if care is accessed from other providers and/or a test is performed.
- Develop an electronic interface with mobile health devices for patients to notify the practice regarding key patient data, such as weight gain for a patient with congestive heart failure.
- Educate patients on what to do if they are ill or have questions after office hours.
- Institute 24/7 secure, electronic access for patients, such as to a nurse triage unit or physician on call.
- Institute telehealth visits with chronic care patients to add touch points to supplement or replace the face-to-face visit.
- Proactively communicate with patients who have been seen in the emergency department or discharged from the hospital

and other facilities within 24 hours. If clinically appropriate, schedule face-to-face appointments.

- Develop effective methods for members of the care team to consult one another; for example, a primary care physician (PCP) may have questions about a patient with diabetes; in lieu of sending the patient to be seen, the PCP would have access to speak or consult with the endocrinologist to determine the appropriate action to take. E-consults have been embraced by many providers, especially if the communication can be facilitated immediately.

These actions not only reduce inbound call demand, but they also provide outreach support to patients that is initiated by the practice, rather than the patient. Indeed, these actions migrate the practice into the new era of healthcare delivery—proactively managing the care of the patient, instead of simply waiting for the patient to call.

Post-procedure and postoperative patients

For patients who have had a procedure or operation performed, there are many questions that arise. Anticipate those questions and proactively provide answers in writing or video format (see previous section), but also recognize that the event creates anxiety and discomfort for the patient and his or her caregivers. It's not uncommon for practice staff to be irritated or even upset with patients who call about their postoperative care. The pertinent information, in the minds of the practice's employees, was communicated during the office encounter and the patient should have remembered it. The fact is that patients—most people, in fact—retain only a fraction of what you tell them, particularly if you don't reinforce it with the information in writing. Of course, the situation is made only more challenging by the fact that many patients are inherently anxious even if the procedure is routine. It's vital to recognize that the procedure is only routine for your practice, not the patient.

Consider the following action to reduce inbound call demand and anticipate the needs of post-procedure and post-operative patients:

- Focus on the transition of care. Schedule the postoperative visit at the time of scheduling the procedure or surgery. If discharge dates are variable, add the protocol of scheduling the postoperative visit to the patient's discharge process. Proactively communicate with the discharge planner, social worker, care coordinator, or the family to discuss the patient's needs, as opposed to waiting for the patient to call.
- Communicate with patients upon their discharge from the surgery center, hospital, emergency department or other healthcare facility. Assign staff to call or securely message patients before and after scheduled procedures or operations to check on their welfare and seek out any questions they may have. Proactively providing the patient with a list of common questions and answers regarding their procedure or surgery may avoid an inbound telephone call to ask routine questions. As we discussed in Chapter 4, analyze the reasons for inbound calls and develop web-based information and other tools to provide to patients in order to assist them in better understanding their care. At minimum, communicate with patients within 24 hours of their discharge to evaluate their medical condition (if clinically appropriate). Schedule the follow-up appointment during that outbound communication. This ensures that every patient who is discharged is sent home with follow-up appointment information in hand or is contacted within a defined period after discharge.
- Supplement verbal instructions with written tools. Provide instructions on paper or in electronic form, to include video, and review the information with patients before they leave. Or, give patients a notepad and pen to make notes of your instructions. Patients should be encouraged to write your instructions down on the notepad, or on their smart phones, iPads, or laptop computers. The patient needs to not only "hear" the communication, but also internalize and interpret

the information through active listening, which reading and note-taking can help accomplish.

- Solicit questions from patients. During or at the end of the appointment, ask patients if they have questions about their visit and the care they are receiving. Too often patients are ushered out hastily after appointments. The few minutes you save by not prolonging the office encounter are used many times over in handling patients' communications and messages later on. The physician may play this role, and his or her efforts may be supplemented by a health coach or patient navigator assigned this role.

You won't eliminate all patient follow-up telephone calls, nor should that be your goal, as it's important for patients to call if they are having a problem. However, being proactive can help you and your patients.

BEST PRACTICE

IF YOU WANT PATIENTS, AS WELL AS THEIR FAMILY MEMBERS AND CAREGIVERS, TO REMEMBER VERBAL INSTRUCTIONS AND INFORMATION, GIVE THEM A NOTEPAD AND PEN WITH WHICH TO WRITE IT DOWN; ENCOURAGE THEM TO MAKE NOTES ON THEIR IPAD OR OTHER PORTABLE DEVICE; OR GIVE THEM THE INFORMATION IN WRITING.

Billing

A significant volume of inbound calls for many medical practices is due to patients calling with billing questions. These communications, which often result in payment, are critical to manage efficiently and effectively. You may have a patient who wants to figure out a way to pay you and just needs clarification regarding his or her bill, but becomes frustrated with your telephone system. You, therefore, are not getting paid. Head off these problems by developing strategies to better manage billing-related telephone calls.

- Evaluate your billing statements. Take the time to review your billing statements to see if you can prevent some of the calls. Your statement might read, "insurance pending." You know that means you've sent a claim to the patient's insurance company, but the patient could be left with the impression that his or her insurance coverage may be in jeopardy. Misinterpreting that to mean that their insurance coverage is "pending," confused patients call to seek clarification. That's not the only source of confusion—complex terms like "contractual adjustment" or basic ones like "applied to deductible" may leave the patient befuddled. If you can't understand your own statements or realize that they could easily be incorrectly interpreted, rest assured that your patients may be having the same problems—and therefore aren't paying. Revising statements for better clarity reduces the number of information-seeking, noncollection telephone calls to business office staff—and helps you redirect staff time to improving collections.

- Create direct access to your business office. Give your business office a direct telephone number, or route an option in the ACD directly to the business office. Print those numbers on billing statements so patients can call them directly. Set up a communication function on your website or patient portal to improve access to your business office staff.

- Collect at the point of care. By expanding patient collections at the time of service (for example, collecting patients' out-of-pocket payment responsibility prior to elective procedures provided your contracts permit), you can minimize the volume of statements sent to patients, and respond to patients regarding their questions about their bills while they are in the office rather than via a telephone call.

- Establish secure, electronic statements to patients and encourage queries about billing questions to be made electronically—and online bill payment. When a billing question is received online, the business office has the opportunity to research and respond to the patient's concern rather than simply take a message and get back to the patient after the account is researched. Inbound billing calls are expensive for your practice; each costs an estimated $4.50 to resolve.[2]

Improving the process related to billing calls can result not only in cost savings, but also the opportunity to improve collections for your practice.

General information
While the areas that we have reviewed certainly constitute a significant portion of your calls, there are myriad other reasons for which patients call, including patients seeking general information regarding your practice. Take action to reduce or eliminate general information calls. Here are some steps to consider for your practice:

- Provide a comprehensive website supplemented by a brochure highlighting key information. Make sure your website and brochure include the general information that patients need to access your practice. They should incorporate a detailed description of your practice, including services, hours of operation, financial policies, directions, and so forth. The time that your staff spends on the telephone with new patients who need directions to the practice can be reduced by instructing patients to go to your website. Include a map with driving and parking directions in the languages that accommodate your patient population. Inaccurate directions produce late patients or cause them to become totally lost and miss their appointments altogether. Be sure to have several people unfamiliar with your location test your driving directions before posting them. And don't forget to include information about public transportation, where applicable.

- Optimize your social media presence. Increasingly, patients are interacting with social media, such as Facebook and LinkedIn, to learn valuable information about your medical practice. Establish a Facebook page and/or LinkedIn profile for your practice. Consider a Twitter handle, or other social media options that may be popular for your patients. Having a social media presence allows you to better serve patients, and they won't need to call you as often.

- Integrate forms with your website and/or patient portal. Integrate common requests for information from patients, such as medical records requests, to allow patients to "self-serve." Also, use your website to obtain information you need from patients, such as registration and medical history forms that need to be completed prior to their visit.

Determine what other needs may be met by proactively providing patients with information. Your patients benefit by making the information readily available, and your practice benefits by reducing inbound calls for general information requests.

Hours of operation

Regardless of the type of call, being able to respond to calls during the business day is vital to maintain patient access—and your practice's bottom line. Although it was historically acceptable to limit inbound telephone calls to several hours in the morning and afternoon, practices today recognize the negative impact that these restrictions place on their patients and referring physicians. In addition to the access limitations, transferring callers to an answering service or routing them to voicemail at lunch or any other time of the day simply batches and delays work. Thus, it actually consumes more time to manage telephones in a restricted environment, which is certainly not the intention. Answer your telephones starting a minimum of 30 minutes before your office hours begin, and keep your telephones open at lunch. These time periods are essential to capture the needs of patients and referring physicians, who often need to call you before they begin their workday or during their lunch period.

BEST PRACTICE

ANSWER YOUR TELEPHONES STARTING A MINIMUM OF 30 MINUTES BEFORE YOUR OFFICE HOURS BEGIN, AND KEEP YOUR TELEPHONES OPEN AT LUNCH.

Getting the basics down—'Who's on Deck?'

Patients call for so many reasons that locating the correct staff member who can manage the call can be a chore. Give each telephone operator a daily list of everyone's responsibilities (unless it's inherent in their job title) and whereabouts. Distribute the list on paper, write it on a white board each morning in a central location in the practice, set it to be the practice's screen saver, and/or reside it on the practice's intranet. Regardless of how it is executed, the few minutes it takes each morning to prepare this "who's on deck?" communication saves precious time in looking for someone to answer a patient's question. It also lessens the caller's time on hold. Similarly, you can extend these protocols to work processes by establishing a knowledge center for your practice. Place scripting tools and practice resources on a searchable intranet or other secure, password protected website to ensure that employees have the tools they need at their fingertips to assist callers.

Converting Inbound Calls to Outbound Calls

In our discussion, we have provided examples of turning an inbound call to an outbound call. You might wonder why these recommendations are made: isn't a call just a call regardless of how it is generated? The current focus of telephone management for practices is, most commonly, handling inbound calls. Inbound call traffic, on which we've come to rely for most of our patient telephone contacts, is more difficult to handle than outbound traffic. To understand why, consider four facts:

- First, a call requires synchronous communication. In sum, the caller and the person who can respond to the call must be available at the exact same time. Because staff members are not sitting idle waiting for calls to be directed to them, they are most often not readily available—or they are totally unavailable—when an inbound call is received and processed. It's often not possible for a practice to handle an inbound call immediately, thus initiating the time-consuming—and expensive—process of taking a message, performing the action dictated by the patient's communication, and, finally, attempting to reach the patient again.
- Second, because the caller is challenged with gaining access to a particular person or a specific area of the practice, the process involves technology to appropriately route the call (automated attendant, combined with an ACD) and/or a live operator(s). Either way, your practice spends a pretty penny just to handle the call—yet often ends up just taking a message.
- Third, inbound calls arrive and cluster during times that also happen to be peak volume times for office encounters. Thus, rarely can resources be matched with the work—the call—without a significant opportunity cost.
- Fourth, the inbound calls must typically be processed blindly—when the call is received, staff must ask questions of the caller to pull a paper record or query an electronic record to determine the proper context of the call. Either way, there's a time delay and a cost to understanding the context of the call (and importantly, documenting it). Many practices have an EHR system; however, the staff member taking the call must take the time to review the information, determine the context, and decide to whom the message must be routed.

When the call can be anticipated or the context determined before the patient calls you, the four challenges of the inbound call are significantly diminished. Although it still requires time, an outbound call permits the task to be performed at a lower cost because a message need not be generated or distributed. Furthermore, there is confirmation that the resource at the practice (the person with the requisite knowledge to manage the call) is actually available. Finally, the calls can be made during times when there is a lower workload in the practice.

So, how can an inbound call be replaced with an outbound call? By coordinating the care of your patients. Place an outbound call (or other form of communication) before and after a procedure or surgery; proactively contact patients immediately after receiving their test results; follow up with patients who just received surprising information; query your registry for patients who have uncontrolled chronic illnesses and provide opportunities to coach them; and recall patients for missed encounters based on your recommended clinical guidelines.

This is not to discount the challenge of reaching the patient, but consider that most patients now carry portable cellular phones. If you don't make any outbound calls, your patients will surely call you. Furthermore, by initiating a communication that does not rely on the telephone—for example, your patient portal—you oversee the mode of communication. A proactive approach to communication puts your practice in charge, allowing you to determine what method works best for your practice.

Get started on turning more inbound into outbound communication; it's more efficient and it reduces the need for patients to call your practice.

BEST PRACTICE

OUTBOUND COMMUNICATION IS MORE EFFICIENT BECAUSE YOU'RE IN CONTROL OF THE WORK; AN INBOUND CALL CONTROLS YOU.

Reducing Inbound Calls

In addition to reducing the inbound calls based on the reasons for the calls, there are opportunities that can reduce inbound call volume regardless of the nature of the call. These opportunities include leveraging technology, reducing rework by initiating a "virtual" encounter, discouraging unnecessary inbound calls, and decreasing transfers. Let's take a look at each of these opportunities.

Leverage technology

Evaluate the calls that you are receiving, and determine if there are alternative forms of communication. For example, the offices of referring physicians may be calling to request a consultation. Instead of handling the process over the telephone, create a secure, automated request process that prompts the referring physician to provide the information you need to assess the appropriateness of the referral and/or make an appointment for the patient. Alternatively, engage with the health information exchange in your community to facilitate the referral process—and streamline post-visit communication as well.

As another example, leverage your patient portal by expanding services and information available to patients via the web. Clinical and business access options available to patients online are outlined in Exhibit 5.5.

In many cases, patients who interact with your portal conduct the work that your telephone operators and triage staff have traditionally performed in the past. When patients use the portal, they are responsible for accurately identifying themselves (no more finding the "right" Mary Smith; the patient has a unique user identification and password); routing their request to the appropriate party by determining their own needs (appointment request, for example); and documenting their own message. Converting inbound telephone calls to secure, electronic messages, routing requests via the patient portal, and migrating inbound scheduling calls to self-scheduling leverages technology to improve access and minimize inbound telephone calls—and save your practice both time and money.

Adopt virtual encounters

Some of the activity that occurs on the telephones represents an excellent example of rework—performing and managing the same work over and over again—in a practice. Rework is not only inefficient, it's expensive. Do the work—and do it right the first time. To reduce rework, incorporate the idea of a "virtual" encounter into each physician's schedule. A virtual encounter is essentially a "meeting" with paperwork (note that this concept differs from a virtual visit with a patient that constitutes an encounter performed via telehealth). "Paperwork" is a general term used to describe the inbound work that may be physically on paper, but may also be in electronic form. For the latter, these are often called "tasks" that typically present to the provider via his or her EHR system's work queue.

[EXHIBIT 5.5] Online access options

Clinical Access	Business Access
• Online scheduling	• History/billing forms
• E-consults/visits	• Health risk assessment
• Telehealth/mobile health	• Survey instruments
• Secure e-mail messaging	• Bill pay
• Test results reporting	• General information
• 3D virtual experience	

Embracing this concept, the physician sees patient 1, then patient 2, then patient 3, and then attends to his or her "in-box," thereby addressing work—in paper or electronic form—after every third patient. This virtual encounter involves spending a few minutes to review the messages and tasks that have been received since the last virtual encounter, regardless of the form that they take. Typically, a formal time is not reserved on the schedule for this work; however, by instituting this approach and formalizing the support role of staff to help make it work, the physician can manage forms, messages, and other tasks more effectively and better meet patient access demand.

> **BEST PRACTICE**
>
> DO THE WORK - AND DO THE WORK RIGHT THE FIRST TIME.

The efficacy of this strategy tends to fall off dramatically if the virtual encounter isn't performed at least once an hour, primarily because the volume of inbound work is too significant to handle in a timely manner unless it is handled in small batches. Moreover, the success of this virtual encounter hinges on the physician's support staff to accurately and comprehensively document, as well as prioritize, messages and tasks. The physician's inbox should include any outstanding messages that need response, required documentation that needs to be completed, or other pending tasks. When physicians perform this virtual encounter several times during a clinic session, work is completed throughout the day and very little of it remains at day's end.

If you make the virtual encounter concept part of each physician's day, you reduce the amount of recall and rework time that is now likely part of his or her evening ritual after the office closes. It puts an end to patients calling your practice multiple times due to frustration with your response times. The virtual encounter also increases staff efficiency—employees spend far less time recording, filing, batching, and organizing messages and related paperwork.

> **BEST PRACTICE**
>
> MAKE A VIRTUAL ENCOUNTER PART OF EACH PHYSICIAN'S DAY TO ATTEND TO TELEPHONE MESSAGES, THEREBY ENSURING A QUICK TURNAROUND TIME TO THE CALLER—AND AVOIDING REPEAT CALLS TO THE MEDICAL PRACTICE.

Don't just assume that this virtual encounter is solely the responsibility of the physician or advanced practice provider, however. Before a message is incorporated into the provider's inbox, the operator must inquire of the caller: "Is there anything that I can do to help you?" If a message is necessary, support staff must be trained to take a comprehensive message, clearly outlining the nature of the communication. Furthermore, the contact information of the caller should be accurate. Most importantly, when the provider offers a response, the clinical support staff must take timely and appropriate action.

> **BEST PRACTICE**
>
> BEFORE A MESSAGE IS TAKEN, THE OPERATOR SHOULD INQUIRE OF THE CALLER: "IS THERE ANYTHING THAT I CAN DO TO HELP YOU?"

If the virtual encounter isn't an option for your practice, consider requesting the nurse or medical assistant to formally "check in" with the physician every few hours to review messages that need to be addressed. Quickly review them with the provider when he or she is between patients. This method of working is certainly acceptable—the key is to pull in the work.

By attacking the work before it attacks you, you allow your staff the opportunity to better help your patients—and efficiently and effectively support the provider as he or she sees patients.

Don't encourage unnecessary inbound calls

Examine whether you are encouraging unnecessary telephone calls via your behavior. For example, instructing the patient to "call to let us know how you are doing" may sound customer friendly at the time, but when the patient calls in the midst of a busy Monday morning to inform you that she had a lovely weekend, that instruction does not have its intended effect. On Monday morning, employees answering calls are busy on the telephones and clinical staff members are occupied with patients, thus creating a situation in which the patient's call may not be received in the manner the patient expected. Don't be frustrated with patients who make this seemingly unnecessary call: you asked the patient to call and the patient is only doing what you instructed.

Examine the reasons for inbound telephone calls and determine if you are encouraging unnecessary telephone calls; there may be a better way for patients to obtain information or supply information you need rather than resort to the telephone.

Decrease transfers

Transferring the call throughout the practice is a costly, time-consuming process, and one that can frustrate the patient. Develop internal protocols to limit or collapse the number of telephone transfers that take place between practice staff simply to resolve the telephone call. Route callers to someone who has the knowledge and skill to respond to the caller in a one-call, one-touch fashion. In addition to the staff time, every transfer is wasted time for the patient, and it ties up the line for the next patient. Staff your telephones with employees who can help the patient—or route callers to employees who have the requisite knowledge to respond to the caller with the accurate answer, thereby eliminating the many inefficiencies of playing "pass the caller."

BEST PRACTICE

STAFF YOUR TELEPHONES WITH EMPLOYEES WHO HAVE THE REQUISITE KNOWLEDGE TO HELP THE CALLER, THEREBY ELIMINATING THE INEFFICIENCIES ASSOCIATED WITH 'PASS THE CALLER.'

Summary

Evaluate the reasons for inbound calls to your practice and create an action plan to improve call management. Instead of hiring more telephone operators or adding telephone lines to try and make telephone problems go away, look for ways to redesign your patient flow processes related to the reasons for your inbound telephone calls. Work to transition an inbound telephone call to an outbound telephone call, thereby taking control of the telephone process and ensuring that the caller's request is handled by the most appropriate staff member—the person who has the knowledge required to respond to the caller and get the job done, the first time. Finally, explore the steps you can take to reduce inbound call volume.

Establish your telephone system and the processes around it so that patients can access your practice by pulling the value they seek and getting information they need without having to resort to a telephone call. Patients don't want to be mired in a long trek through your telephone system any more than you want to spend all that extra time answering avoidable calls to your practice.

End Note

1. Elizabeth W. Woodcock, Front Office Success: How to Satisfy Patients and Boost the Bottom Line (Englewood, Colo.: Medical Group Management Association, 2017). Available at www.mgma.com and www.amazon.com.
2. Deborah Walker Keegan and Elizabeth W. Woodcock, The Physician Billing Process: Navigating Potholes on the Road to Getting Paid (Englewood, Colo.: Medical Group Management Association, 2016). Available at www.mgma.com and www.amazon.com.

[CHAPTER 6]

Telephone Staffing

It is important to not only hire the right type of staff for the telephones, but also to ensure that you have the right volume and skill mix of staff for effective patient access management. Importantly, the work assignments of telephone staff members and the training and resources provided to them lay the groundwork for telephone success.

In this chapter, we discuss the nuances of staffing your telephones to include:

- Recruiting telephone staff;
- The right type, volume, and skill mix of staff members for the telephones;
- Staff work assignments;
- Staff training and resources; and
- Staff performance management.

Although there are ways to decrease your call volume, there will always be telephone calls to a medical practice—and there must be people to answer them. The key is to ensure that you have the right number of people with the right skill mix to effectively manage your telephones.

Recruiting Telephone Staff

Recognizing the importance of the telephones to medical practice success, it is puzzling to see many medical practices delegate the telephones, the vital lifeline to patient access, to the lowest paid, least trained, and, often, least experienced staff members. In addition to redesigning the "what" and "how" of handling the telephones, be sure to look carefully at who you hire (or have hired) to answer the telephones. The employee who answers your telephone represents your patients' first "moment of truth" with your practice, and determines whether patients' questions or concerns are routed to the correct party. This employee, often referred to as a telephone operator, is usually the individual who also schedules an appointment on behalf of the patient. Indeed, the schedule defines the execution of your practice's most precious asset—your providers' time. Investing in this critical position cannot be overlooked or underestimated.

Telephone operators need knowledge of medical practice operations and must possess customer service skills. Many medical practices are staffing their telephone operations with employees who have clinical training. With clinical knowledge, staff can follow your protocols to ask appropriate follow-up questions that ensure a complete message is taken, as well as determine the type of patient visit and urgency of the visit that is needed.

BEST PRACTICE

YOUR TELEPHONE OPERATOR REPRESENTS THE PATIENT'S FIRST IMPRESSION OF YOUR PRACTICE. MAKE SURE THE EMPLOYEE HAS THE KNOWLEDGE AND SKILLS TO MANAGE A HIGH VOLUME OF CALLS WITH QUALITY AND COMPASSION.

Pre-employment assessment
Having the right staff starts with hiring the right staff. Consideration should be given to including "tests" in the hiring process. (See Exhibit 6.1 for a sample pre-employment questionnaire.) Spelling, grammar, clinical terminology, telephone management, and similar tools to assess the candidate should be considered to improve hiring selections. When you find the right candidate, request a working interview. Typically a paid half- or full-day, this "interview"—also referred to as a "job shadow"—is a chance for the candidate to understand the job by actually experiencing it, and it allows the practice to assess the candidate outside of a formal job interview.

> **[EXHIBIT 6.1]**   Pre-employment questionnaire
>
> 1. [Evaluation of candidate's service orientation and effectiveness.] When a patient calls, what would you suggest as the initial greeting?
> 2. [Evaluation of ability for candidate to take a comprehensive, legible message.] Please take a message based on this information. "Hi, my name is Susie. I'm calling on behalf of my elderly mother. She was seen by one of your doctors early last year and has had some recurring issues in her left knee. She has limited transportation available to her and would like to make an appointment for the morning of November 7th to see Dr. Smith. Is he available and what information can be completed ahead of time?"
> 3. [Evaluation of grammar skills.] Please review the following message, and identify the mistakes that you see. (Provide the message to the candidate.) *Judy Jones (DOB 6/23/76) called today with questions about her medicatin. She developed a rash on her toursoe, and is having troubel swallowing food. The last doos of medicine she took was yesterday mrning. She kneads to speak with someone twoday. Please call her this even ing at 404.555.1211.*
> 4. [Evaluation of ability to multitask. When taking calls, you are on a headset talking while simultaneously typing messages. A patient calls with a convoluted insurance question that you don't understand. You must both take the message and respond to the patient according to the policies and procedures from the insurance handbook; however, you are not able to locate the answer in the handbook. How do you handle this situation?
> 5. [Evaluation of ability to cope with change.] Three weeks after you start and having been extensively trained on the telephone system, the practice upgrades to a new telephone system that you find difficult to learn. How do you handle this change?
> 6. [Evaluation of ability to work under pressure.] Your manager has set a deadline to complete several tasks by the end of your shift. As the deadline approaches, you have just enough time to complete the tasks when you get a call from an irate patient who has been waiting all day to receive a callback from his physician. How do you handle this situation?
> 7. [Evaluation of ability to handle difficult situations.] You are assisting a patient with an immediate need when two additional calls come in at the same time. How do you handle this situation?
> 8. [Evaluation of ability to deal with challenges.] A patient calls and is very upset. He becomes more belligerent during the call and begins using profanity directed toward you. How do you respond?
> 9. [Evaluation of teamwork.] How would your (former) peers describe you?
> 10. Which software applications have you used? What products and services have you dealt with? What is the typical call volume you have experienced in a single day?
>
> *(continues)*

> **[EXHIBIT 6.1] Pre-employment questionnaire (continued)**
>
> 11. What do you like most about being a telephone operator? What do you like the least?
> 12. If there was one reason that we should select you over the other applicants, what would that be?
> 13. Why do you want to work for our organization?

BEST PRACTICE

HAVING THE RIGHT STAFF STARTS WITH HIRING THE RIGHT STAFF.

Hiring philosophy

It is rare for a job candidate to have all of the knowledge and skills you require in the role of a telephone operator for a medical practice. The candidates tend to have strong medical practice knowledge and skills–or they have a strong customer service background. With that in mind, determine your philosophy regarding staff hires. Do you want to hire for medical practice knowledge and then educate the new hire to customer service? Or do you want to hire for customer service and then educate the new hire to medical practice knowledge? When it comes to the telephones, many medical practices have elected the second approach—hiring staff with excellent customer service backgrounds and then conducting staff training for medical terminology and medical practice operations.

BEST PRACTICE

MANY MEDICAL PRACTICES HAVE ELECTED TO HIRE STAFF WITH EXCELLENT CUSTOMER SERVICE BACKGROUNDS AND THEN TRAIN FOR MEDICAL TERMINOLOGY AND MEDICAL PRACTICE OPERATIONS.

As medical practices recognize the importance of the telephones to patient access and overall practice success, more innovative staffing models are being adopted to ensure that all staff members have customer service skills, as well as knowledge of medical practice operations. For example, some medical practices employ 'access coordinators' to respond to the telephone, as well as schedule appointments and take messages. Others appoint all staff members as 'clinical associates'—super-trained staff who are able to manage telephones, the front office, and back office clinical support. In these situations, a dual focus on customer service skills and medical practice knowledge ensures that employees have the requisite knowledge to manage all customer-service interactions to a high level.

Identification of candidates

Most practices rely on placing a job advertisement in the local media, contracting with a staffing company, or asking existing staff to help identify candidates to aid in the search for a new employee. Besides these traditional hiring methods, practices are finding success with identifying candidates via online sites like Monster.com and Indeed.com. LinkedIn is also an excellent source for posting information about your new position.

Of course, a background check is a necessity for all employees today. Consult with an attorney regarding opportunities to evaluate the backgrounds of your candidates.

BEST PRACTICE

USE SOCIAL MEDIA TO IDENTIFY CANDIDATES AND TO EVALUATE THE CANDIDATE'S FIT WITH YOUR MEDICAL PRACTICE.

Creating a Telephone Staffing Model

Forget trying to staff your telephones based on how many physicians each employee serves. The number of employees you need depends on how many telephone calls need to be answered, and the level of service you want to provide. Telephone call volume fluctuates by day and by time of day, hence the requirement to create a flexible staffing model rather than a static model. If a medical practice assigns the same number of staff members to the telephones regardless of call volume, the telephones will likely be either over- or understaffed.

To build the staffing model for telephones, use the data you captured in Chapter 4: Call Demand and Performance. This included: (1) inbound call volume by day of week, (2) inbound call volume by time of day, and (3) inbound call volume by reason for call. The first two measures are useful in determining the number of staff members you need to assign to the telephones in your practice. The third measure—inbound telephone calls by reason for call—helps you determine the skill mix you need for staffing your telephones. For example, a high volume of clinical calls may signal the need to establish a telephone nurse triage unit for your medical practice. As discussed in further detail below, your practice should also account for the desired level of timeliness and quality of the telephone communications when staffing the telephones. The more employees the practice deploys to answer the telephone, the higher the performance in terms of abandonment rate, average speed to answer and service level. It's important to recognize, however, that a balance of these elements is critical. While an additional hire may improve the abandonment rate, ASA and/or service level by a percentage or a second—that small, incremental improvement may not justify a $30,000 (or more) annual investment. Indeed, staffing telephones is not a one-time decision, but rather an ongoing monitoring of both quantity and quality to balance the cost of the operation with the desired outcome in terms of caller experience.

BEST PRACTICE

TO DETERMINE THE NUMBER OF STAFF MEMBERS YOU NEED TO MANAGE YOUR TELEPHONES, USE STAFF WORKLOAD RANGES. BE SURE TO ALSO ACCOUNT FOR THE DESIRED LEVEL OF WORK QUALITY YOU EXPECT FROM YOUR TELEPHONE STAFF.

To determine the number of staff members needed to manage inbound telephone calls, we first employ expected staff workload ranges. The staff workload ranges depend on patient population, information systems, level of automation, and work processes your practice has embraced. For example, if your staff members are required to gather and/or deliver more information in each call than peer practices, you will have a longer transaction time and therefore should expect staff to work at the lower end of the productivity range. As another example, if your employees have complex telephone processes, they may need more time than staff members in other medical practices to perform their work, again suggesting the low end of the workload range.

Given these influencing variables, don't just embrace and apply the staff workload ranges. Instead, measure the time it takes your staff to handle each type of telephone call, compute an average handle time, and apply that handle time to reach your practice's ideal workload range.

Based on average transaction times, the workload ranges for telephone staff are reported in Exhibit 6.2.

Exhibit 6.3 demonstrates a method to identify the volume of staff needed to manage the telephones, accounting for the variation in arrival rates of the calls by day of week. This method uses data from the medical practice regarding the inbound calls and the staff workload ranges expected of telephone operators. In this exhibit, the number of scheduling calls and the number of calls that require a message to be taken is reflected for each day of the week (Monday through Friday). The expected staff workload range is then reported for each day based on the type of call—scheduling vs. message-taking. With this data in hand, the practice can simply do the math: Divide the number of calls by the workload that is expected to arrive at the number of staff full-time equivalents (FTEs) needed to manage the telephones.

As demonstrated in Exhibit 6.3, 2.50 staff FTEs are needed to manage scheduling calls on Monday and only .50 FTE is required for Friday.

[EXHIBIT 6.2] Workload ranges for telephone staff

The following workload ranges are expected from staff involved in call management, based on average transaction times.*

Practice Operations Task	Workload Range
Telephones with messaging	300 to 500 calls per day
Telephones with routing	1,000 to 1,200 calls per day
Appointment scheduling with mini-registration	75 to 125 calls per day
Appointment scheduling with full registration	50 to 75 calls per day
Nurse triage	65 to 85 calls per day

*The workload range depends on patient population, information system, level of automation, and work processes used at the practice. The workload ranges have been built assuming a seven-hour productive day with one staff member performing this function full time.

Source: Woodcock, Elizabeth W. 2017. Mastering Patient Flow. Reprinted with permission from the Medical Group Management Association, 104 Inverness Terrace East, Englewood, Colorado 80112. 877.ASK.MGMA, www.MGMA.com.

Similarly, 1.25 staff FTEs are required to take messages on Monday, reducing to .25 FTE on Friday. This exercise helps to evaluate the volume of staff you have assigned to your telephones to make sure it is linked to the actual work that needs to be performed, recognizing that the work varies by day of week. To refine your staffing analysis, measure and assess data based on hours per day. As discussed below and in Chapter 7, the workload associated with telephones can vary significantly, so staffing strategies that include part-time or temporary staff are commonly used by today's medical practices.

Accounting for quality

Although staffing based on these quantitative data regarding the transactions is important, be sure to consider the level of service you expect to deliver to patients and referring physicians who call. Because

[EXHIBIT 6.3] Staffing the telephones

	Monday	Tuesday	Wednesday	Thursday	Friday
Scheduling calls	250	200	150	100	50
• *Staff expectation*	*100*	*100*	*100*	*100*	*100*
• Required staff FTE	2.50	2.00	1.50	1.00	.50
Message calls	500	400	300	200	100
• *Staff expectation*	*400*	*400*	*400*	*400*	*400*
• Required staff FTE	1.25	1.00	.75	.50	.25

the arrival of calls is sporadic, it is essential to develop a staffing plan that accounts for the transactions represented by the calls, as well as the level of service desired by the practice. Use the quality indicators presented in Chapter 4 and the more detailed telephone management strategies outlined in Chapter 5 to refine your staffing model. Because the arrival times of calls varies throughout the day, in general, a practice may need to employ more staff than the workload range data alone would suggest to meet or exceed the desired level of quality. Before adding staff, however, recognize that other initiatives, to include changing the demand for calls, should be deployed.

Employee downtime

A warning about staffing your telephones: employees who answer the telephones, like all of us, have a tendency to pace their work to match the demands of the moment. Let's look at a case study of this scenario in action to see the impact it has on telephone work in the medical practice.

◆ CASE STUDY ◆

Orthopaedic Surgery Associates

ORTHOPAEDIC SURGERY ASSOCIATES (OSA), A BUSY ORTHOPAEDIC SURGERY PRACTICE, LOOKED FOR WAYS TO REDUCE STAFF. DURING ITS TELEPHONE ANALYSIS, OSA REALIZED THAT THE VOLUME OF INCOMING TELEPHONE CALLS WAS MUCH GREATER ON MONDAYS, THEN DECREASED AS THE WEEK WENT ON. HOWEVER, ON FRIDAYS, EVEN THOUGH THE CALL VOLUME WAS LOWER, THE OPERATORS' TIME ON THE TELEPHONE WAS HIGHER PER CALL. THE OPERATORS SPENT 25 PERCENT MORE TIME PER CALL ON FRIDAYS BECAUSE THEY EXPANDED THEIR EFFORTS TO MATCH THE DEMANDS OF THE MOMENT.

This is a natural phenomenon, but it's often hidden. Even the manager of OSA thought that the practice needed another operator. Rather than hire another operator, however, consider the following actions:

- Share this data with your telephone staff so they see their work pace, and trend this over time so they can see their fluctuating call times; and
- Don't let this "Friday pace of practice" lead you to unnecessarily increase overhead; instead staff for the work.

In this case, rather than hiring additional telephone staff for the entire week, OSA hired a part-time staff member to work on Mondays, effectively staffing for the work.

Estimate your staffing needs based on how you have configured your telephone operations and the workload ranges listed in Exhibit 6.2. Don't take the workload ranges at pure face value—if an operator must walk from his or her desk to deliver every message to the nurses' station, for example, then adjust the expected workload range to reflect the additional time for this courier function.

Staff skill mix

Now that you have the volume of telephone staff needed by day (and, upon further refinement, by hour of day), it's time to identify the skill mix you require to successfully staff your telephones. To perform this analysis, use the data you gleaned in Chapter 4 when you measured your telephones related to the reason for inbound call to determine your volume of clinical-related calls and your volume of business-related calls.

Clinical calls require knowledge of medical issues to respond to the patient, which may involve decisions about triage, advice, prescriptions, test results, or other similar clinical issues. Business calls are those that relate to scheduling, general questions, billing, referrals, and other nonclinical issues for the medical practice. Armed with this data, you can work to align your staffing skill mix needs to meet the patient inbound call demand by type of call. Use the workload ranges outlined previously in Exhibit 6.2 to build the number of staff needed to manage the telephones based on type of call—clinical or business—while accounting for the work quality you expect to be delivered. The following case study provides an example of this approach.

Refine these data based on day of week and time of day to develop the staffing model needed to manage your inbound call demand. Next, consider the level of quality that you expect to deliver, noting that high levels of quality typically require additional staffing rather than relying exclusively on the estimates derived based on volume.

It is also important to review the inbound call volume and abandonment rates in "real time" to redeploy staff as appropriate to manage peak demand. If, for example, a higher volume of calls than typically received is coming into the practice, additional staff may be needed for defined time periods or the practice may need to assign another employee(s) to

> ### ◆ CASE STUDY ◆
> #### Family Medicine Associates
>
> FAMILY MEDICINE ASSOCIATES (FMA) RECEIVES 500 INBOUND CALLS PER DAY. LET'S ASSUME THAT FMA CAPTURED THE REASONS FOR THESE CALLS AND LEARNED THAT HALF OF THE CALLS ARE FOR CLINICAL ISSUES AND HALF ARE FOR BUSINESS ISSUES, WITH HALF OF THE BUSINESS CALLS INVOLVING SCHEDULING AND HALF INVOLVING MESSAGE-TAKING. FMA USES THE STAFF WORKLOAD RANGE BENCHMARKS REPORTED IN EXHIBIT 6.2 TO BUILD ITS STAFFING MODEL.
>
> CLINICAL CALLS: INBOUND CLINICAL CALLS TOTAL 250. DIVIDE 250 BY THE BENCHMARK OF 65 TO 85 CALLS PER DAY FOR NURSE TRIAGE TO DETERMINE THAT YOU NEED 2.94 TO 3.85 FTE STAFF TO MANAGE CLINICAL CALLS.
>
> BUSINESS CALLS: INBOUND BUSINESS CALLS TOTAL 250, WITH 125 FOR SCHEDULING AND 125 FOR MESSAGE-TAKING. DIVIDE 125 BY THE BENCHMARK OF 300 TO 500 CALLS PER DAY FOR MESSAGE-TAKING TO DETERMINE THAT YOUR STAFFING NEED IS .25 TO .42 FTEs TO MANAGE THE MESSAGE-TAKING CALLS. THEN DIVIDE 125 BY THE BENCHMARK OF 50 TO 75 CALLS PER DAY FOR SCHEDULING WITH FULL REGISTRATION TO DETERMINE YOUR STAFFING NEED OF 1.67 TO 2.50 FTEs TO MANAGE THE SCHEDULING CALLS. ADDING THESE TOGETHER, FMA RECOGNIZES THAT IT NEEDS 1.92 TO 2.92 FTE STAFF (ROUNDED TO 2.00 TO 3.00 FTE STAFF) TO MEET ITS CURRENT INBOUND BUSINESS CALL DEMAND, NOTING THAT IT RECOGNIZES THE NEED TO MONITOR ITS PERFORMANCE AS EXPRESSED BY ABANDONMENT RATE, AVERAGE SPEED TO ANSWER AND SERVICE LEVEL TO ENSURE THAT IT IS MEETING ITS EXPECTATIONS REGARDING THE EXPERIENCE OF ITS CALLERS.

log into the telephones to assist with management of inbound calls. The goal should be to meet the expected performance standards while still providing quality service to patients, referring physicians, and other callers.

Staging the Telephones

Get the telephones "off stage" to separate the work of the face-to-face visit from that of the telephones. In this manner, front office staff members either arrive and exit patients or they are assigned to the telephones, not both. Telephone work should not be performed in front of patients who are arriving to or departing from the practice.

BEST PRACTICE

GET THE TELEPHONES "OFF STAGE," SEPARATING THE WORK OF THE TELEPHONES FROM THE FACE-TO-FACE VISIT WITH THE PATIENT.

Similarly, clinical staff members either support the visit itself or are assigned telephone responsibilities (and increasingly, virtual medicine responsibilities such as handling secure, electronic messaging with patients). That is, nurses or other clinical staff members are assigned to assist with the face-to-face patient visit or are assigned to work on communication, not generally both roles. In this fashion, the employees are fully devoted to their respective work tasks. By concentrating the work, one nurse is able to manage the communication of two to five providers (depending on the volume of communication), thus centralizing this role within the medical practice or within a pod or suite of physicians. The alternative would be for each nurse to assume responsibilities for communication throughout the day in addition to their face-to-face time with the provider and patient. Intermixing communication and face-to-face responsibilities is a sure-fire prescription for less than optimum performance in both areas, particularly given the new and expanded roles for clinical support staff to support the requirements associated with accountable care, pay-for-performance, value-based and medical home models of care.

Regardless of where the operators (or those assigned to telephone duties) are located, provide these staff members with cordless headsets so they can be mobile as they talk with callers and to improve ergonomics related to telephone work.

Staff Education

One of the best ways to educate staff to handle telephones is to assign a high-performing staff member to provide on-site training support. Most telephone systems permit additional staff—a high-performing staff member and new hire, in this case—to listen in to calls. After hands-on system training, have the new hire spend up to a week listening, watching, and learning from the high-performing staff member. Then reverse roles with the current staff member observing the new hire as he or she responds to patient inquiries.

Discontinue training at peak call volume periods to permit the current staff members to be fully deployed in their work. During these periods, the new hires may be assigned to review scripting, conduct role playing with the manager, and other similar work that furthers their orientation and training to the job.

If resources allow, assign a staff member to perform quality assurance (QA) audits and training. This involves sampling telephone calls (if recorded), work that stems from telephone calls (for example, registration, scheduling, and message-taking), and other qualitative measures. The QA auditor/trainer may be tasked to work especially with new staff members; however, routine audits of all telephone staff are recommended. (See Chapter 7 for further discussion about quality related to staffing.)

During periods of low call volume, rotate the new telephone staff to the clinical area to observe patient flow. This rotation should be limited to one or two hours at a time, with the staff member assigned to "shadow" a nurse or medical assistant who is handling inbound clinical calls. This exposure enhances the fund of knowledge of telephone operators and improves their decision-making and judgment skills as they respond to patient inquiries.

BEST PRACTICE

DURING PERIODS OF LOW CALL VOLUME, ROTATE NEW TELEPHONE STAFF TO THE CLINICAL AREA TO OBSERVE PATIENT FLOW AND "SHADOW" A NURSE TO IMPROVE KNOWLEDGE AND DECISION-MAKING SKILLS.

Be sure to train a select group of additional employees to manage the telephones so they can work when telephone operators and nurse triage telephone staff are on vacation, out ill, or taking an extended leave. Consider the use of per diem staff who can be called in on short notice to work the telephones during unplanned staff absences.

Develop an education and training program that goes beyond policies and procedures and encompasses more than the knowledge typically gathered during one-on-one operator-to-operator training. For those handling nonclinical calls, this extended training should include some clinical education about common—and not-so-common—reasons for calls, medication questions, and handling urgent issues. Task the manager with leading staff in role-playing exercises, joint meetings with nursing and front office staff regarding call management, and discussions of required reading from articles or other materials. (See Chapter 7 for a discussion regarding the development of a knowledge center to be used for successfully managing scheduling protocols.)

It is essential that you clearly outline, in writing, clinical calls that must be immediately escalated because they require clinical judgment. These escalated calls should not trigger a response from the operator (unless he or she has the appropriate clinical training), but rather signal a circumvention of the standard message-taking protocol and an immediate need for someone on the clinical team to handle the call. It is recommended that a nurse coordinator, physician, and medical director, in that order, be assigned the 'next-call' responsibility so that escalated calls never go unhandled. Guidance to determine calls that should be escalated, and the methods by which these calls should be handled, must be incorporated in staff training.

For all staff assigned the responsibility of managing telephone calls, as well as physicians, advanced practice providers, nurses, and the many other persons who may answer a call, training on the telephone system itself is important. In addition to answering a call, include training about establishing and checking voicemails (if applicable) and how to appropriately transfer a call.

Staff Resources

Among the many steps you can take to optimize the telephone in your medical practice, an important one not to overlook is gathering feedback from your staff. Learning how to meet staff needs to do a better job can produce notable improvements in productivity, as well as in job satisfaction and reduced employee turnover. Try these actions:

- Improve the working conditions for your telephone staff. Discuss equipment needs with staff members. Do they need hands-free, wireless headsets? Better chairs? Height-adjustable desks? You may avoid future Workers' Compensation claims by paying attention to ergonomics and buying quality equipment.

- Discuss information needs with staff members. Do they need access to instant messaging to alert the triage nurse that a patient is calling again? Is the EHR system available to them to inform the caller whether a task such as test result notification has been completed? Do they need a training update on the EHR system? Do they need access to the "on-call" list for communication from the hospital? Determine what resources you can deliver to your telephone staff to improve their effectiveness.

- Share telephone data with the telephone operators and triage nurses so they can see the volume of inbound calls they manage, abandonment rates, time on the call, and other similar data. This knowledge permits them to self-manage and work to meet the performance expectations you have defined for telephone work.

Your employees are a wealth of resources. At minimum, on an annual basis, ask each staff member: "What is the one thing that I can get for you to help you do your job better?" You'll be surprised—often pleasantly—about their responses.

> **BEST PRACTICE**
>
> At least once a year, ask each employee: "What is the one thing that I can get for you to help you do your job better?"

Staff Performance Management

Institute a formal performance management process for telephone staff. The process should be incorporated into daily or weekly feedback for new employees, as well as bi-annual performance reviews for seasoned employees.

- Review performance expectations and data with all staff as they relate to volume and quality. On a routine basis, share these telephone statistics with the staff.

- Evaluate both the quantity of calls and quality of work of the staff involved in call management by listening to recorded calls (if applicable), sampling messages, reviewing the quality of responses and service to patients, and evaluating the turnaround time to respond to messages.

- Hold joint meetings with telephone and practice staff to review call data, scripting, and impact to scheduling. These meetings can also be a forum to clarify protocols, suggest changes to current policies and procedures, and handle other similar

issues so that all recognize their role in meeting the needs of patients.
- Hold staff accountable for meeting service standards (see Chapter 11 for recommended telephone service standards).

Managing the performance of your staff is critical to ensuring that your telephone operations are optimized. You can have the best technology in the world, but you must have the right people with the right knowledge and skills to be successful.

Summary

Staffing the telephones with an appropriate compliment of staff, trained with the right skills, is a prerequisite for telephone success. The employees who answer your telephones are a direct reflection of your practice's access. These staff members often have more touches with patients than any other staff in the medical practice. Recruit well and provide the training and resources needed for the staff to function at optimal levels. Take the extra time to fully assimilate these staff members onto your care team.

[CHAPTER 7]

Call Centers

Recognizing the opportunity to gain efficiencies, standardize patient experience, train employees and dedicate management oversight, many medical practices have formed call centers. Depending on the needs of the practice, call centers have been established to focus on key access points of your practice such as appointment scheduling, referrals, patient portal inquiries and support, post-discharge coordination of care, physician-to-physician consult facilitation, prescription renewals—essentially serving as the virtual "front door" to the practice to manage all communication. In these centers, inbound call management and increasingly, outbound call management take place. Managed by a few employees—or hundreds—a call center permits a dedicated investment in technology, space, employees and management to ensure effective communication with the practice.

In this chapter, we explore call centers and help you determine whether it is time to consolidate telephone operations in your medical practice. Whether your practice is large or small, the development of a well-executed call center offers a unique opportunity to showcase the practice's attention to patient and referring physician satisfaction and successfully achieve the goals of improving patient access and service delivery. Recent healthcare trends place additional importance on an intentionally designed call center to efficiently handle a practice's communication.

In this chapter, you will learn the various aspects of a call center, which include:

- The definition of a call center;
- Key decision steps in call center formation;

- How to staff a call center;
- Workforce efficiency;
- Designing a call center; and
- Best practices in call center management.

What Is a Call Center?

A call center is a group of employees, typically co-located in the same physical space, who are focused on appropriately and efficiently handling the telephone calls of an organization. Alternative names that are being embraced by medical practices include "contact center" and "access center." Although telephone staff members have historically been referred to as "switchboard operators" or "agents," call center employees are increasingly being referred to as "patient navigators," "patient service representatives," and "access coordinators." These titles reflect the importance of the call center to the practice and its stakeholders.

The scope of a call center has no boundaries. There is no minimum number of staff members required to constitute a call center; it's not uncommon to have a call center staffed by three employees—or more than 300. There are no specifics on the size or specialty of the medical practice; practices with just a few physicians—or those with hundreds of physicians—can institute and operate a successful call center. Furthermore, there is no definition of the type of calls that the call center handles. In a medical practice, a center can focus on incoming telephone calls only, or a mixture of incoming and outgoing calls. Moreover, the call center may handle all calls—clinical, registration, insurance, referrals, and scheduling, as well as billing—or just one of these functions. Referring physicians may be the only callers routed to the call center, patients may be the sole focus, or calls managed by the call center may be a combination of both. Finally, the nature of the call center varies. A call center can serve as a switchboard operation using employees to distribute calls to the appropriate party or it can manage the full gamut of callers' needs—a 'one call does it all' approach, staffed with schedulers, nurses and medical assistants. Although the designation "call center" may be simple, the structure, composition, and staffing of the center are far from elementary.

Why begin the journey of exploring a call center for your practice? When patients or referring physicians communicate with your practice, they expect to receive a consistent and standard experience; however, as various employees throughout the practice answer calls, this standard experience is difficult to implement and enforce. Practices can use various tools and scripts that target employees; however, enforcing consistency and providing the standard experience across numerous positions and extensions are difficult to achieve. Challenges have become more evident in recent years with the increasing complexity of the registration process. Inaccurate information about a patient's demographics or insurance information lead to payment issues. Indeed, almost any inaccuracy results in no payment.

A call center offers the opportunity to consolidate this initial contact within the practice, allowing one group of dedicated employees who have received focused training and reinforcement to handle calls with a consistent approach and experience for the caller. Furthermore, these employees are held accountable for their performance. For a call center, success is typically measured via its ability to manage the volume at the expected level of quality. Although there are dozens of measurements associated with quality, the ones most often used by call centers are abandonment rate, average speed to answer and service level. (See Chapter 4 for a discussion of these and various other quality measures associated with telephone operations.)

BEST PRACTICE

A CALL CENTER OFFERS THE OPPORTUNITY TO CONSOLIDATE THE INITIAL CONTACT WITH THE PRACTICE TO A GROUP OF DEDICATED STAFF WITH FOCUSED TRAINING. MEASURE THE QUALITY OF THE CALL CENTER BY ITS SERVICE LEVEL. SERVICE LEVEL IS THE PERCENTAGE OF CALLS THAT ARE ANSWERED WITHIN A PRE-DEFINED WAIT THRESHOLD.

Appropriately responding to the call is just the beginning. Many practices have staff members who have large, diverse workloads. For staff members who are tasked with serving the needs of physicians, nurses, and patients being seen in the office, picking up the telephone is not always a priority. Thus, the use of voicemail is very high in these scenarios, and response times to callers are often very poor.

In sum, when telephones are under everyone's purview, they are often no one's responsibility.

In addition to dedicated staff, focused oversight and management can be beneficial. When calls are distributed to extensions throughout the practice, it is difficult to specify an individual who has primary responsibility for how the calls are handled and the service is delivered. Decentralized call models are often managed by leaders who are also charged with additional responsibilities for front office, revenue cycle functions, and clinical support, to name a few. In contrast, a call center offers direct oversight concentrated on managing communication with patients and/or referring physicians. This focused expertise is critical in managing telephone-based interactions that are not as controlled as patient arrivals at a front office. As every practice knows, calls do not come into the queue consistently throughout the day; they can be sporadic and difficult to predict, and the reasons for inbound calls are diverse. The potential to successfully and cost-effectively allocate and manage staff resources while maintaining superior levels of quality is what a dedicated call center can deliver.

In this chapter, we focus primarily on responding and processing telephone calls; however, in today's environment, a call center is no longer limited to focusing on communicating via the telephone. Communication methods now include electronic messaging, chat, and social media, all of which need to be considered when developing the communication approach of the practice and the potential role of the call center in managing these new methods. Call centers are increasingly serving the role of processing referrals and transitions of care, often working from task lists or work queues to facilitate communication with patients. Other roles include prescription renewals, portal support questions—and still others. Furthermore, the call center can formulate the infrastructure for outbound call campaigns for communication related to preventive services, post-discharge care management, and other recommended care.

Thus, call centers are being leveraged to handle incoming calls, as well as outbound communication. Regardless of the method of contact, awareness regarding regulatory issues that may impact communication is vital.

BEST PRACTICE

> THE RECOGNITION THAT WHEN TELEPHONES ARE UNDER EVERYONE'S PURVIEW, THEY ARE OFTEN NO ONE'S RESPONSIBILITY.

Key Decision Steps in Call Center Development

As part of your overall communications strategy and to gain a better understanding of the discussion that follows, let's explore some key considerations to determine if a call center is the right solution for your medical practice.

Current quality

First, assess your current level of quality related to your response time and handling of telephones. Use the tools in Chapter 4 to measure your telephones and compare your current state with your service expectations. Determine your ability to process calls by measuring the percentage of calls that are abandoned, and those that are handled within a certain, pre-determined time period (for example, 80 percent within 30 seconds). In addition, analyze your average speed to answer. Not only does poor performance represent a service improvement opportunity, but it may signal a risk management issue as well.

In addition to measuring these data and others regarding the quality of your telephone operations as derived from your telephone system, consider querying your callers. That is, ask patients and referring physicians for feedback regarding your telephone operations. Hearing the "voice of the customer" is often the ideal way to determine if it is the right time to embark on a call center for your practice. The voice of the customer can also help to convince internal stakeholders that a change is needed. If your current performance falls below your expectations—or those of your callers—consider a call center to provide improved focus and service to telephone management.

Current staffing levels

Second, evaluate your current staffing levels and compare them to staffing workload ranges, as demonstrated in Chapter 6. For staffing in a call center, a key indicator is the "auxiliary time" for operators. Often referred to as "aux time," this is the portion of the work day in which an operator is not available for inbound calls. Measuring aux time—and ideally, requiring the operator to demarcate the reason for the aux time—allows management to understand the burden of work associated with non-call activities. Answering calls for a medical practice is not a simple process, so some level of non-call activity time is warranted. However, this is an area of opportunity if gains in efficiency can be achieved by limiting or reducing the transaction time associated with non-call activities.

If your telephones are over- or understaffed, whether that task is focused or just one of many jobs for an employee, it may be time to consider a consolidated unit to manage your telephones. The training costs and time required to educate new staff regarding telephone management may be repetitive for your practice. A central unit is able to mitigate the service variation due to staff turnover, absences, or departures by having a central, core team focused on the telephones.

Reasons for inbound calls

As a third step in the assessment process for a call center, evaluate the reasons for inbound telephone calls to your practice. Use the tools in Chapter 4 to obtain the reasons for inbound calls to your practice. Exhibit 7.1 highlights key functions often served by a call center, but there is no need to be constrained in your approach. A call center may receive calls from referring physicians as well as calls from patients related to scheduling, triage and advice, general information requests, medical records requests, prescription renewals, test results, or other issues. By assessing the reasons for inbound calls, you are in a position to determine if call consolidation makes sense for your practice.

Delegated authority to manage calls

Next, identify the optimal action you would want call center staff to take when responding to the inbound telephone calls if you had a call center. As depicted in Exhibit 7.2, for example, the action for a physician-to-physician call for this medical practice is for call center staff to have the knowledge and tools to either connect the physicians directly or send the referring physician to the on-call physician. As another example from Exhibit 7.2, if a patient calls to schedule or

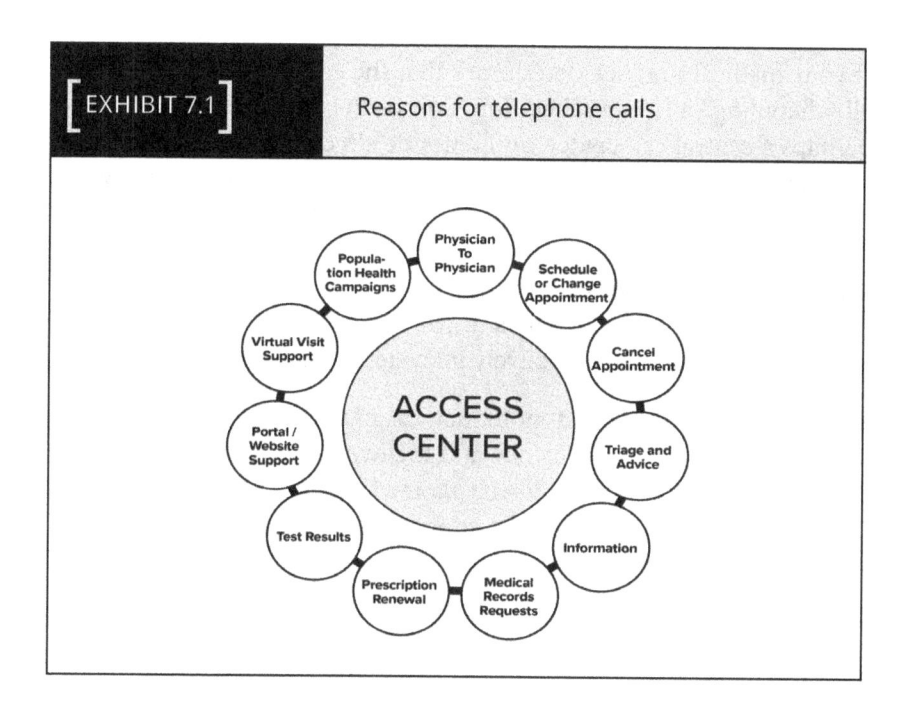

[EXHIBIT 7.1] Reasons for telephone calls

Access Center surrounded by: Physician To Physician, Schedule or Change Appointment, Cancel Appointment, Triage and Advice, Information, Medical Records Requests, Prescription Renewal, Test Results, Portal / Website Support, Virtual Visit Support, Population Health Campaigns

change an appointment, the practice would want its call center staff to be able to make or change an appointment directly, not simply transfer the caller to a scheduler. Evaluate the reasons for your inbound calls and determine the delegated authority you would want to provide to the call center. If a decision is made to form a call center incorporate these protocols into your practice management system, or create a knowledge guide that can be searched and referenced by staff members electronically.

BEST PRACTICE

To determine if a call center will benefit your practice, evaluate the current quality of your telephones and the current staffing levels to ascertain the magnitude of improvement opportunity. Then outline the delegated authority you would want to provide to the call center staff to manage the key reasons for inbound calls. This will help you assess the need for a consolidated call center operation.

If your medical practice determines that the call center must transfer all scheduling calls to a scheduling unit or the physician's nurse, then perhaps a central call center would not be effective in your practice. It may serve as only another step or barrier for patients who simply want to make an appointment to see you. However, if many of the calls can be handled by call center staff as opposed to being redirected to practice staff, then a call center can provide economies of scale for telephone work. The practice can also benefit from consolidating the knowledge and expertise needed to effectively manage inbound call demand.

A call center offers great potential to add specific strategies that improve both practice efficiency and the overall patient experience. If the transition to a call center is well planned with intentionally designed processes, the structure of a call center offers advantages that cannot be achieved by other systems.

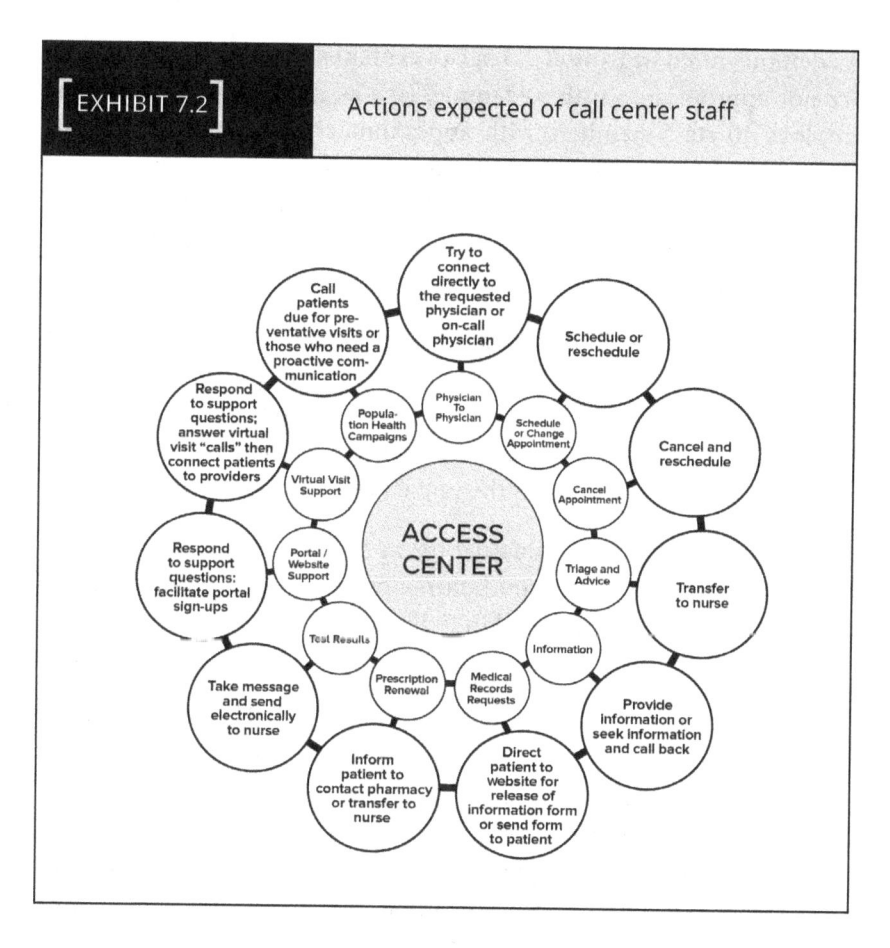

[EXHIBIT 7.2] Actions expected of call center staff

Centered on **ACCESS CENTER**, with surrounding categories and associated actions:

- **Physician To Physician** — Try to connect directly to the requested physician or on-call physician
- **Schedule or Change Appointment** — Schedule or reschedule
- **Cancel Appointment** — Cancel and reschedule
- **Triage and Advice** — Transfer to nurse
- **Information** — Provide information or seek information and call back
- **Medical Records Requests** — Direct patient to website for release of information form or send form to patient
- **Prescription Renewal** — Inform patient to contact pharmacy or transfer to nurse
- **Test Results** — Take message and send electronically to nurse
- **Portal / Website Support** — Respond to support questions; facilitate portal sign-ups
- **Virtual Visit Support** — Respond to support questions; answer virtual visit "calls" then connect patients to providers
- **Population Health Campaigns** — Call patients due for preventative visits or those who need a proactive communication

Staffing a Call Center

Since staffing is often one of the key considerations in implementing a consolidated center, let's explore how to staff a call center and the impact of quality related to staffing. As discussed previously, call centers have the potential to provide a more consistent level of quality to patients by allowing the practice to dedicate a specific structure to prioritize the telephones and provide oversight by management. All of these benefits can be eroded if the call center does not have—and maintain—an appropriate number of employees. The quantity of inbound and outbound calls, as well as the quality of telephone management, must be constantly analyzed.

As demonstrated in Exhibit 7.3, a call center can falter if staffing levels are not appropriate. In this example, let's assume that the call center employs 10 staff members with approximately 12,000 inbound calls per month, but two employees decide to leave. Staff attrition impacts quality quickly. Quality, as measured by service level in this example, falls from an acceptable 82 percent of calls answered within 30 seconds to less than 60 percent with the loss of the two staff members.

In addition to staff fluctuations, a key management issue for call centers is to evaluate and handle the variation of incoming calls. There is no appointment schedule for telephone calls; inbound calls are scattered throughout the day and the week. Call centers are challenged to predict these fluctuations and address the impact in a cost-effective manner.

Exhibit 7.4 highlights the fluctuation in volume by day of the week in one practice. Calls also vary by time of day, further complicating a staffing model as demonstrated in Exhibit 7.5.

If all patient calls are equally important—whether they arrive Monday, Wednesday, or Friday, or at 8:00 a.m. or noon—then the goal is to ensure consistently positive service throughout the week, as well as the day. Without a clear staffing strategy, call centers will not have enough employees to handle peak volumes, which causes quality to plunge, or they have too many employees, which is expensive and may leave an excess of non-value-added downtime. Adding the responsibility of outbound calls may enhance the complexity, however, the inclusion of outbound call responsibilities may reduce downtime, if applicable.

Forecasting call volumes

To mitigate problems from inappropriate staffing, it's important to develop a formal staffing model for your call center. At minimum, you need to acknowledge the call volumes you expect. This is always an interesting exercise that combines both science and art as you attempt to predict future volumes based on information from the past. It's important to recognize associated non-call work (i.e., "aux time"), as this may vary by type of call. Fortunately, there are several call models to explore that help align your specific volumes with the staff needed

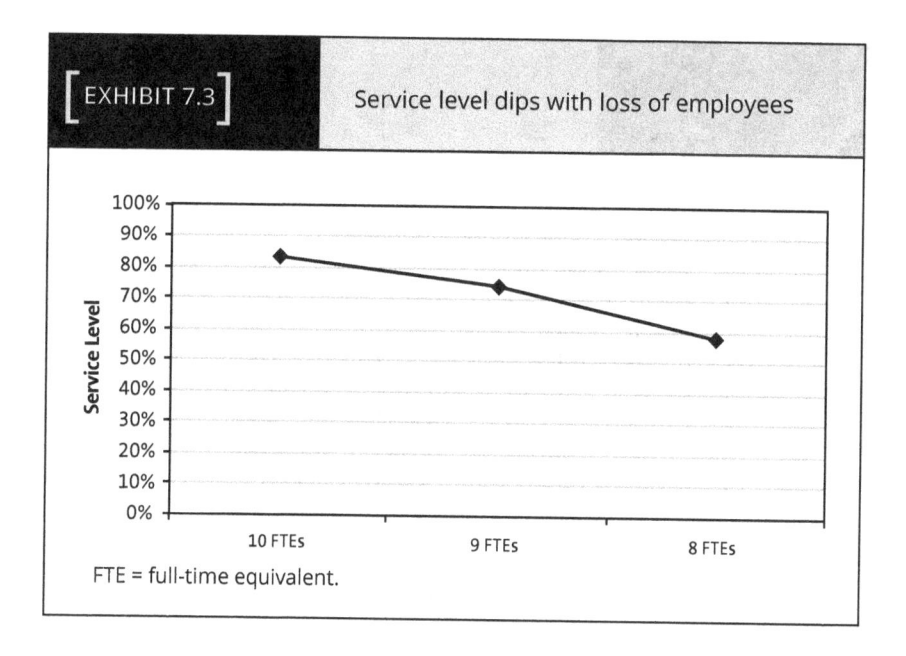

[**EXHIBIT 7.3**] Service level dips with loss of employees

[Line chart showing Service Level on y-axis (0%–100%) versus FTEs on x-axis. Data points: 10 FTEs ≈ 83%, 9 FTEs ≈ 73%, 8 FTEs ≈ 55%.]

FTE = full-time equivalent.

to meet a targeted level of quality. In this section, we present three models—from very basic to sophisticated—to consider when factoring your practice's staffing needs.

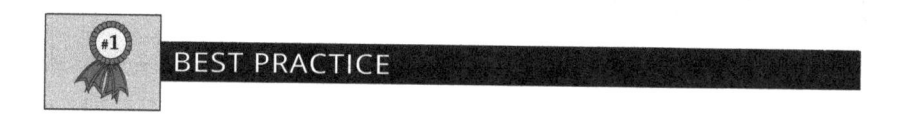

BEST PRACTICE

TO DETERMINE THE APPROPRIATE STAFFING MODEL FOR YOUR CALL CENTER, USE BASIC FORECASTING, THE ERLANG C METHOD, AND/OR WORKFORCE MANAGEMENT TOOLS. THE GOAL IS TO DEVELOP A STAFFING MODEL ALIGNED WITH BOTH CALL VOLUMES AND QUALITY EXPECTATIONS.

Basic forecast

A nontechnical method can be used to produce a rudimentary forecast model for staffing a call center. The following three items are needed to calculate this model. This model is similar to the staffing example we

[EXHIBIT 7.4] Weekly inbound call demand by day of week

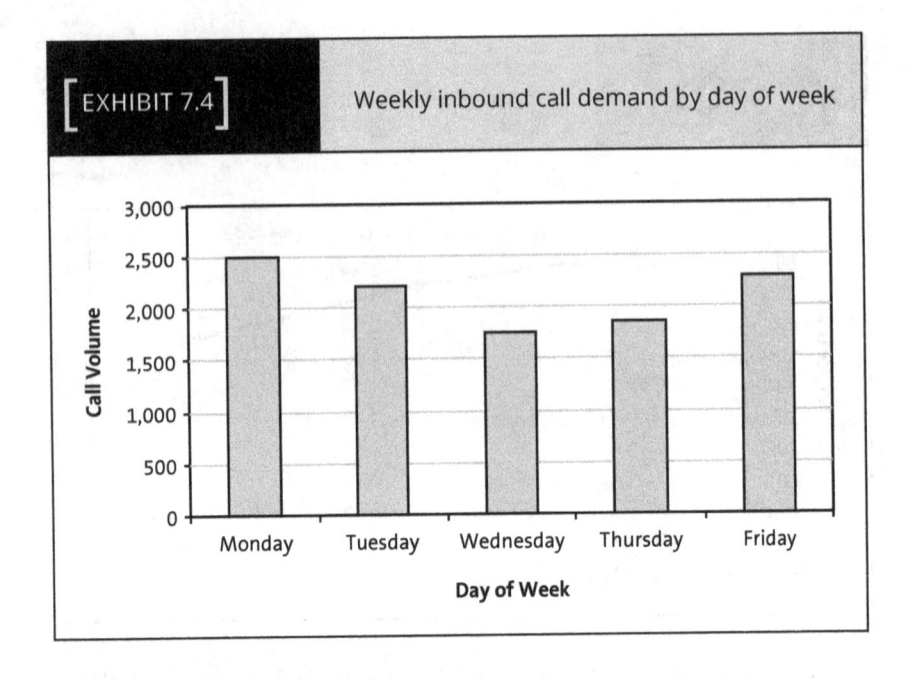

Day of Week	Call Volume
Monday	~2,500
Tuesday	~2,250
Wednesday	~1,800
Thursday	~1,900
Friday	~2,350

[EXHIBIT 7.5] Inbound call demand by time of day

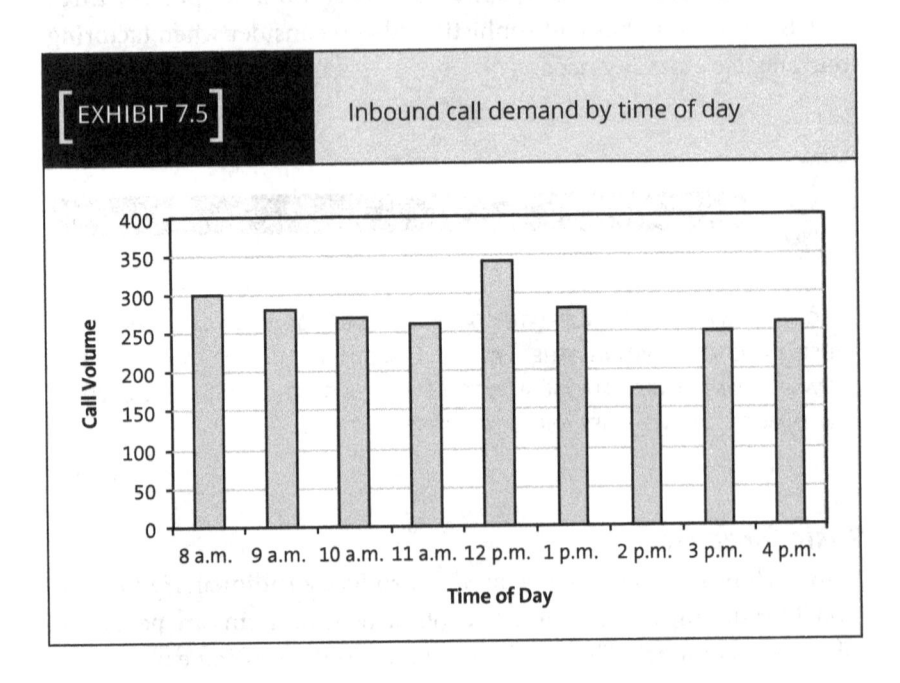

Time of Day	Call Volume
8 a.m.	~300
9 a.m.	~285
10 a.m.	~275
11 a.m.	~265
12 p.m.	~350
1 p.m.	~290
2 p.m.	~185
3 p.m.	~260
4 p.m.	~270

provided in Chapter 6. Although it would be ideal to measure this over a significant period of time, we recommend an evaluation timeframe of at least one month.

1. **Call volume:** The volume of calls by day of week and time of day can usually be obtained from the telephone system. This provides basic data to understand the volume of calls handled by the practice. (For example, in assessing inbound calls, 75 calls are received by the practice on Mondays between 8 a.m. and 9 a.m.)

2. **Call type:** Ask staff members who manage your primary telephone extension to use manual tick-mark sheets to provide a rough breakdown of the types of calls received by the practice. This allows you to estimate the volume of incoming calls by type of call.

3. **Average duration:** Finally, determine the average call duration, which is referred to as "talk time" or the "handle time" for telephone operations, associated with each type of call. As this is often not readily available, it may require conducting a time study. For example, your average scheduling call may consume 4.5 minutes. It's important to account for any necessary post-call work associated with the function, which may require adjusting the handle time to achieve the actual duration required for the task.

Focusing on the examples presented above, let's assume the practice receives 38 calls related to scheduling on Monday morning between 8:00 a.m. and 9:00 a.m. Each scheduling call takes an average of 4.5 minutes to complete; therefore, the total minutes needed during this hour to answer these calls is 171 minutes of work. Dividing that time by the 60 minutes that constitutes an hour, 2.85 FTEs (full-time equivalents) are required. You would need to repeat this calculation for each call type and hour of day to arrive at your overall hourly staffing plan, keeping in mind that this basic calculation does not account for employee downtime or the variation in call arrival. Because it is limited to data regarding incoming call volume and duration, the model does not take quality into consideration. Therefore, if this staffing model is embraced, we recommend that the staff estimates be rounded upward. The 2.85 FTEs in this example should be translated into 3.00 FTEs. After staff members have been assigned, quality must be monitored carefully to ensure that the number of employees who have been deployed are adequate, as it is not uncommon for this model to underestimate the staff required to maintain a base of satisfied callers. If outbound call activities are also included, these would need to be considered in the calculation in order to effectively deploy staff.

Erlang C method

The second method to staff a call center is one of the most widely used models today for forecasting call center staffing levels for incoming call handling. It derives its name from A.K. Erlang, a Danish engineer who developed the original queuing and trafficking theory. The equation that formulates the method dubbed Erlang C, which is presented below, accounts for call volume and duration, as well as quality.

$$P_W = \frac{\frac{A^N}{N!}\frac{N}{N-A}}{\left(\sum_{i=0}^{N-1}\frac{A^i}{i!}\right) + \frac{A^N}{N!}\frac{N}{N-A}}$$

Where:
- P_W is the probability that a customer has to wait for service
- A is the total traffic offered in units of erlangs
- N is the number of servers

We could write an entire chapter on the meaning of each letter and symbol, as well as how to use this formula. Don't worry; we won't launch into a detailed explanation. Instead, we recommend that you use an Internet search engine to query "Erlang C." In your search, you will uncover a list of websites that offer an Erlang C calculator where you can enter key data as inputs and the formula is automatically calculated for you. Expect to enter call volume and duration, recognizing that it is important to factor appropriate "aux time" into the equation as this is time your staff require to complete the task at hand. The third input is the desired service level. Changing the service level alters the output, which is the number of employees needed to handle the call volume and call duration at the desired service level.

There are two key assumptions to be aware of when using the Erlang C method:

1. Erlang C assumes that the rate of incoming calls is consistent over the defined period, which results in the inability of the model to account for the impact of the variation of call arrivals often experienced with a call center.

2. Erlang C assumes that calls unable to reach a live operator remain in the queue until answered; calls are not abandoned or blocked by the system. Thus, the model does not account for caller behavior.

Despite these drawbacks, Erlang C is still a very useful (and free!) tool in determining staffing needs, as it is readily available and simple to use.

Workforce management tools

The third method for staffing a call center involves workforce management tools. Vendors in the call center market offer workforce management tools as a stand-alone program or a package coupled with other features. These are very powerful tools because they calculate staffing needs based on a detailed history of calls, including call volume, duration, staff downtime, call arrival patterns, and caller behavior (such as tolerance for hold times before abandoning the call), to a per-minute time period. They can also more accurately predict staffing needs if call handling involves both inbound and outbound calls. Using all of this data, often extracted directly from the telephone system (without the need to monitor, analyze, or input information), a workforce management tool can offer a very accurate snapshot of staff needed by time of day and day of week based on the desired level of quality. See Exhibit 7.6 for a sample hourly forecast of staff based on a workforce management tool.

Workforce efficiency

Determining the number of staff needed at different intervals throughout the day and week is the first step in designing a staffing strategy for a call center. How those resources are applied becomes crucial in maximizing efficiency. Let's review some of the key strategies to apply; some of which can be used by all practices, even in the absence of a call center.

> **BEST PRACTICE**
>
> EMPLOY PART-TIME STAFF TO MEET SERVICE-LEVEL EXPECTATIONS. THIS PERMITS A CALL CENTER TO MAINTAIN A CONSISTENT, HIGH LEVEL OF QUALITY THROUGHOUT THE DAY AT A FRACTION OF THE COST.

Part-time staffing

Part-time employees are a vital asset for telephone operations. Look for parts of the day or week that part-time staff members can be applied to target their efforts and to avoid reductions in the quality of your telephone management. For example, a call center may be able to maintain the level of quality that meets the practice's expectations for most of the day; however, when employees begin taking lunch, even though they are staggered over several hours, poor performance may ensue. See Exhibit 7.7 for a display of data, including the area identified as "Opportunity." As this exhibit demonstrates, incorporating a 10 a.m. to 2 p.m. shift of part-time staff into the practice's call center would greatly improve the overall performance of the calls being handled. Incorporating part-time staff into your strategy essentially allows the practice to eliminate the decline in quality by effectively addressing the problem segment of the day at a fraction of the cost of a full-time employee.

The 10 a.m. to 2 p.m. time frame is an advantageous target because there are typically excellent candidates available to apply for the position. Because of the hours, this opportunity often attracts candidates interested in part-time positions that can accommodate their time with school-aged children. This time period targets the practice's major need, as staffing is usually reduced during this time and call volumes during this period are often high. An alternative solution to part-time staffing is to hire a vendor to take calls after a certain service level is reached, thereby supplementing the call center staffing to ensure quality performance.

BEST PRACTICE

ESTABLISH FIRST-CALL RESOLUTION AS A GOAL AND DEPLOY STRATEGIES TO MAKE THIS GOAL A REALITY FOR YOUR TELEPHONE OPERATION.

Telework

Answering the telephone need not require operators to be physically present in the facility. Call centers are offering operators the option to work from home, referred to as teleworking. Operators perform

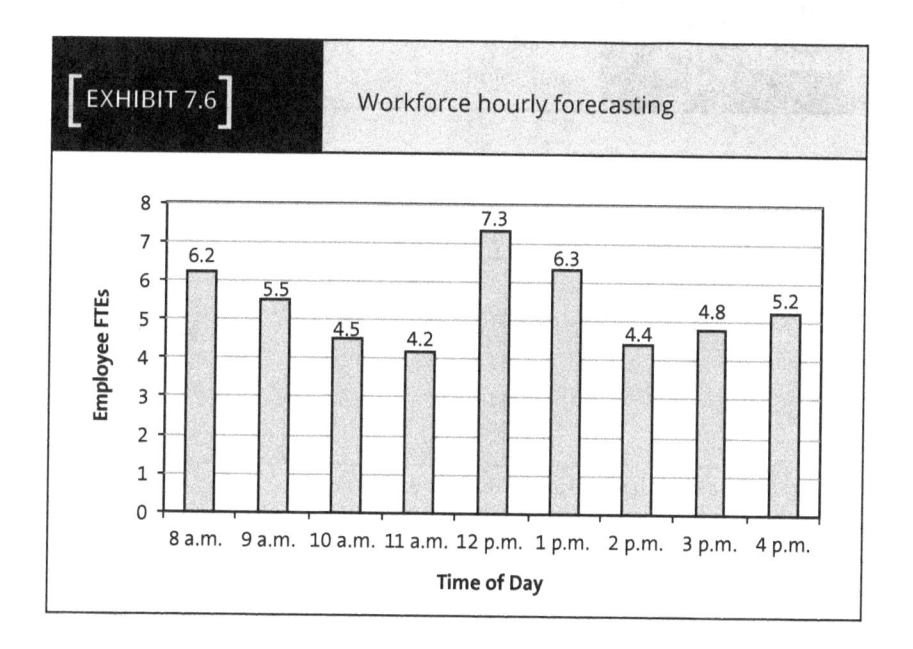

[EXHIBIT 7.6] Workforce hourly forecasting

Time of Day	Employee FTEs
8 a.m.	6.2
9 a.m.	5.5
10 a.m.	4.5
11 a.m.	4.2
12 p.m.	7.3
1 p.m.	6.3
2 p.m.	4.4
3 p.m.	4.8
4 p.m.	5.2

each of the same functions that they would were they sitting at a desk in the call center, but do so from their home. Typically reserved for high-performing employees who have spent a minimum time in call operations at the practice, teleworking offers the following benefits:

1. Improved staff morale;
2. Possible increase in productivity, attendance and performance by operators;
3. Controlled environment with limited distractions for operators;
4. Greater talent pool, particularly if geographical constraints are lifted;
5. Cost savings as it relates to space; and
6. Alternative use of space.

Given the importance of the technology, particularly as it relates to protecting patients' health information, the practice often invests and installs the workstation for the teleworker. The cost of the internet

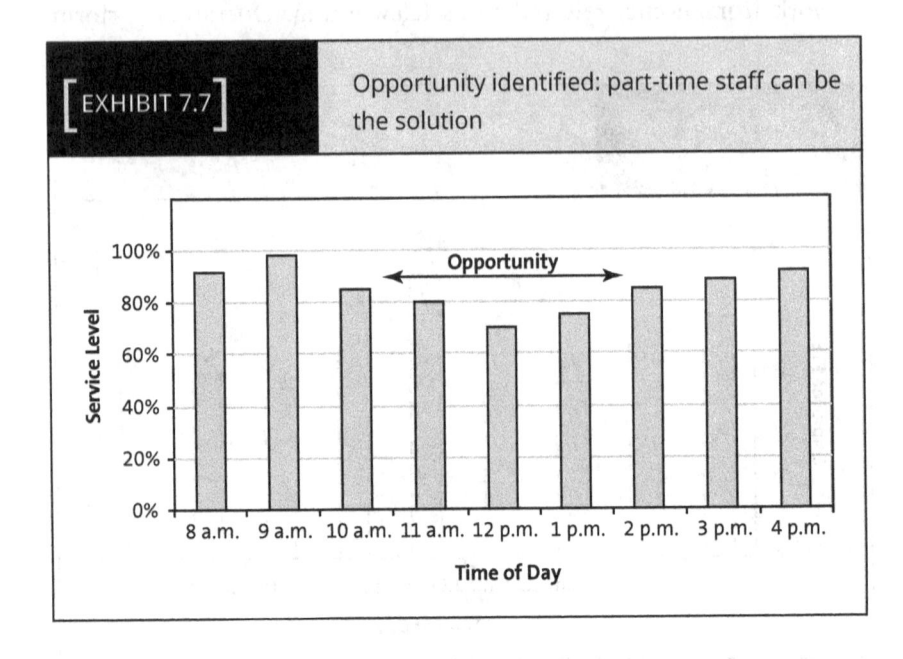

[EXHIBIT 7.7] Opportunity identified: part-time staff can be the solution

connection may be borne by the operator or the practice. Operators are requested to attend staff meetings and training in person and/or virtually. Managers engage with operators via video chats or conference calls, with some call centers requiring a "constant" view of the operator's work area. Teleworking is not for every employee, but offering the option may improve both productivity and performance, while also freeing up space for other use.

First-call resolution

First-call resolution, a concept further discussed in Chapter 9, is the goal for most call centers. Effectively routing the call to the best resource with the knowledge and skill to manage the call is the key to achieving this goal. Since patients call a practice for various needs, the ability to achieve this routing efficiently and effectively can be a challenge. Although there is no single right answer, the following describes four popular options to address first-call resolution:

1. Train staff members to handle the vast majority of calls received by the call center. These must be highly skilled operators who are trained to handle myriad issues. In a large call center, operators may be organized in different "skills" in order to achieve first-call resolution. For example, 100 operators may be organized in five pods of 20 operators with each pod focused on a specialty service line.

2. Deploy a small group of staff members who act as call distributors. These operators answer the call, typically to a so-called "vanity line" (for example, 800-BONES4U) and then quickly distribute these calls to the appropriate party—a specific practice or location, or a designated employee such as a nurse, scheduler, biller, and so forth.

3. Use an automatic call distributor (ACD) that puts the onus on the patient to choose the resource. Through the system, route the call to the appropriate staff member to handle the caller's needs.

4. Create a series of multiple telephone numbers or extensions, or adopt the legacy numbers, that allow callers to be seamlessly

routed to the appropriate staff member, all of whom may be co-located within the same call center.

Evaluate the solution that is best for your practice, based on your telephone system and staff resources, as well as your expectations for call management and quality.

Best agent routing

As you consider how calls are organized, it is important to determine who can best handle the caller's needs. To achieve the goals of a call center—first-call resolution, as well as the desired level of quality—the concept of "best agent routing" is an important consideration.

Best agent routing allows the caller to be routed to the staff member who is best qualified to meet his or her needs. Call centers often refer to this as a "skill." This concept is particularly essential for new staff members who may have been assigned to process a specific type of call but need more time and/or training to handle the call. For a staff member assigned to appointment scheduling, for example, a model may be deployed to route calls from established patients to operators who have one year's experience or less, while more seasoned staff members handle new patient calls. By using best agent routing and ramping up the employee over time, the call center experiences higher first-call resolution and lower hold times. This system also increases first-year satisfaction of the call center by decreasing the learning curve frustration. Although best agent routing is not always possible, discuss the concept with your telephone system vendor to work together to determine how callers can best be routed.

BEST PRACTICE

ADOPT BEST AGENT ROUTING TO LINK THE CALLER TO THE STAFF MEMBER BEST QUALIFIED TO MEET THE CALLER'S NEEDS. THIS HELPS THE CALL CENTER TO HAVE HIGHER FIRST-CALL RESOLUTION AND IT LOWERS HOLD TIMES.

Staff availability

One of the key challenges in handling telephone operations within a call center is to resolve the inevitable fluctuations in staff availability without a noticeable variation in service to the patient. As noted in the previous staff analysis, 171 minutes dictated the need for 2.85 FTEs. However, the reality is that 2.85 FTEs is not actually 171 minutes. Staff members can't handle calls while they are getting a cup of coffee from the break room, using the rest room, receiving training on the new telephone system, or meeting with you to discuss their performance, in addition to the non-call work associated with the communication. Indeed, all of these activities result in time away from answering the telephone. Accounting for standard breaks, the most efficient state of a call center employee is 85 percent productive.

Adding in vacation, sickness, and turnover, this can rapidly fall to 60 percent or less, quickly changing what appears to be a well-staffed call center into a poor-performing one! (See Exhibit 7.8.)

Call centers need to keep such fluctuations in mind and staff accordingly. Staffing options include:

- Employ part-time staff targeted during predictable periods of high call volumes and/or planned absences to minimize any negative impact;
- Use either an external or internal temporary staffing pool to help cover times of need;
- Ask an external vendor to help manage calls when a critical inbound call threshold is reached;
- Engage in outbound or non-call responsibilities; and
- Cross-train practice staff (for example, a medical assistant) to provide temporary telephone coverage.

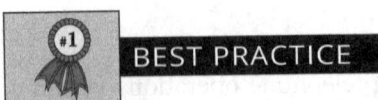

> **BEST PRACTICE**
>
> THE MOST EFFICIENT STATE OF A CALL CENTER EMPLOYEE IS FOR THE EMPLOYEE TO BE 85 PERCENT PRODUCTIVE. MAKE SURE YOUR CALL CENTER STAFF MEETS THIS PRODUCTIVITY THRESHOLD.

Because overstaffing—sinking a significant amount of expenses into the call center—is not a realistic option, the practice must consider the best method to deploy additional staff as needed.

As discussed earlier in this chapter, best agent (i.e., skill-based) routing is a method of grouping the complexity of calls so that the easiest calls can be specifically routed to a staff member or group of employees. With best agent routing, temporary staff, or perhaps even staff members at the practice who are available but typically assigned to other tasks can be assigned to handle the least complex calls. This model allows the call center to manage the call volume at the desired level of quality—at the lowest cost possible.

Call leveling

It is intuitive that there is a variation in the arrival of calls to a medical practice. This fluctuation in volume results in time periods in which there are only a few inbound calls—and moments when the telephone lines are flooded. These times of heavy call volumes are often referred to

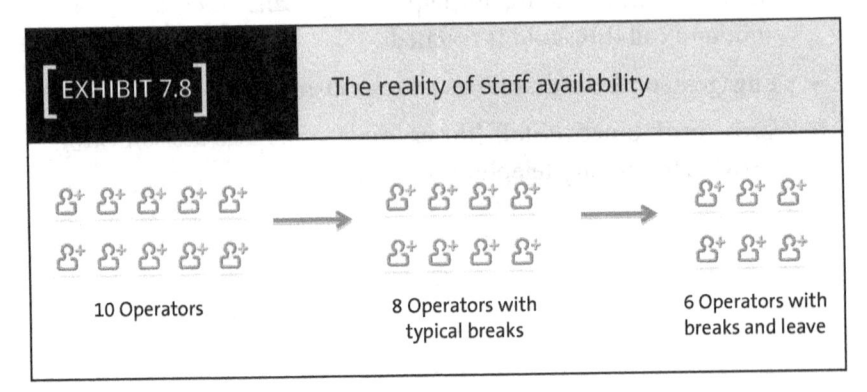

[EXHIBIT 7.8] The reality of staff availability

| 10 Operators | → | 8 Operators with typical breaks | → | 6 Operators with breaks and leave |

as call spikes. Call spikes can cause practices to invest in staff to manage them (who then sit idle during periods of low volume)—or result in low performance in terms of meeting callers' expectations regarding quality. Deploying a strategy to minimize the impact of call spikes on your practice helps to reduce staff costs and improve performance. Focus on "call leveling," also referred to as call shifting—a tactic that features looking for opportunities that transfer workload to times of predictably lower volume.

BEST PRACTICE

> ADOPT CALL LEVELING, SUCH AS A VIRTUAL HOLD SYSTEM, TO LOOK FOR OPPORTUNITIES TO TRANSFER WORK TO TIMES OF PREDICTABLY LOWER VOLUME.

Although it may seem impossible to influence the arrival rate of calls, there are opportunities to shift calls. On the ACD, program an alternative route that is revealed if the hold time exceeds two minutes (or another time period that you determine is best for your callers). This option allows a patient to opt into voicemail and receive a return call within the hour rather than continue to wait on hold.

A similar alternative is to use a "virtual" hold system that features a self-directed callback mechanism. This system is best applied to call centers experiencing heavy call volumes with extended waits in the queue. Patients are provided the option of entering their callback number and exiting out of the call. The call, however, remains in a virtual queue until the call is ready to be handled. When the calls that previously arrived are cleared, the system automatically calls back the patient who is next in line. This is a very useful tool to remove callers' frustration when they are holding in the queue for the next available operator.

For calls with a significant hold time, consider shifting these "overflow" calls to a vendor to answer the call with a live voice and provide the caller with an option to remain in the queue or leave a message for callback. This gives the patient an option if call waits increase. Although all overflow calls can be sent to an external vendor, protocols can be established based on ACD options. For example, clinical calls could be sent to a vendor specializing in nurse triage. The vendor can either resolve the patient's needs or complete a message and transmit it to the internal nursing team for follow-up. Another example is travel directions. These calls are usually time-consuming and most vendors can field these well, or the patient could be directed to a pre-recorded message regarding the practice's location.

As discussed in detail in Chapter 5, reducing the demand for calls by offering alternative communication routes (for example, patient portal or personal health record for medication renewals, appointment requests, and clinical messaging) is the ideal method of call leveling.

Automated appointment scheduling protocols
The task of scheduling appointments for established and new patients is often delegated to the call center in a medical practice. Because the schedule represents the essence of a practice, effectively managing the scheduling process is essential. For many practices, scheduling protocols are recorded in large three-ring binders or on a series of sticky notes that landscape the cubicles of staff members. Not only is it difficult to manage the information in such a format, it is almost always out of date. Automating the scheduling logic is an important factor in reducing the complexity of provider scheduling—and aiding the call center tasked with managing it.

BEST PRACTICE

CREATE A KNOWLEDGE DATABASE. FOR EXAMPLE, AUTOMATE THE SCHEDULING LOGIC AND DEVELOP A SERIES OF QUESTIONS AND SCRIPTS TO HELP CALL CENTER STAFF LINK PATIENTS TO THE APPROPRIATE PROVIDER.

Develop an electronic version of the appointment scheduling protocols to serve as a readily accessible, easily updatable knowledge database. Using the binders and notes to build the reference, create a tool that presents staff with a series of questions and scripts that end with the appropriate physician or provider, as well as the visit type.

Give staff dual monitors, with the practice's practice management system on one monitor and the knowledge database on the other. Or, integrate the database into the scheduling process by embedding the protocols into the practice management system. Your practice may have the internal expertise to develop such a tool itself; if not, vendors (including the scheduling system, if protocols can be embedded) can assist you in creating these protocols. Update the tool regularly to remain accurate. In addition to improving scheduling accuracy, which leads to enhanced revenue, the tool can serve as a resource for staff members regarding ever-changing scheduling protocols. Of course, the knowledge database can be extended beyond scheduling protocols, to include various aspects of the practice's operations that may be useful to all staff and providers.

Quality and training

Most of the strategies we discuss in this chapter are focused on the timeliness of call center staff in answering the telephones. However, once answered, the quality of the call is the determining factor driving satisfaction.

If you develop a call center for your medical practice, institute a quality program focused on adherence to the quality indicators we first described in Chapter 4—including scripting, appropriate tone, call resolution, accuracy, and first-call resolution. To successfully measure performance, the quality program must feature an evaluation of actual calls. Thus, the telephone system must be able to record calls and, ideally, identify them by operator. This technology can be purchased as a stand-alone product or packaged with other software, and may also include speech analytics. The ability to capture and monitor call recordings is essential. When staff members are asked to listen to their interactions with patients after the call has been completed, it is often a very different experience than what they are able to recall. One may also consider purchasing the ability to document the screen itself during the call—often called "screen scraping," in order that the audio may be recorded as well as the specific actions of the staff member that accompanied the verbal exchange.

Although there is no pre-determined volume of calls that must be reviewed, consider a minimum of 10 per staff member per year for a performance evaluation. (Additional call reviews at a more frequent period are recommended, but resource availability must be considered.) Monitored calls should be reviewed with staff members on a timely and consistent basis so that employees can learn from their telephone interactions. Use both positive calls and calls where the staff member has an opportunity for improvement when sharing the calls with staff for performance assessment and improvement.

Call recordings are arguably the best tool for quieting naysayers of the call center, if applicable. By recording 100 percent of calls, the manager of the call center is able to respond to any complaints about service, scheduling errors, or protocols that were perceived not to be followed.

The quality program can be managed and conducted centrally or, for a large operation, decentralized to local supervisory management. The benefits of a central quality program can include unbiased call ratings, as opposed to local management who may instill personal bias in the ratings of the calls. For a busy supervisor, quality monitoring often loses its priority. Also, central quality monitoring offers consistent scoring that is difficult to achieve in a decentralized environment. If the program is decentralized, calibrate quality with reviewers to ensure that quality scores are comparative across managers.

To ensure success, couple the quality program with a comprehensive training program. Centralized and consistent training is a key benefit to the call center. When employees are trained together and work alongside one another, they can rely on each other to reinforce the training without adapting other practices. Training can be conducted in waves during business hours or it can include all staff members in training after business hours. If the training is focusing on a new process or tackling cultural competency issues, for example, after-hours training is preferred so that the group can learn and interact together. If training focuses on processes or is related to specific tasks, then a wave approach can work well. A well-rounded training program not only engages with staff members on or near their hire date, but also offers ongoing and consistent training throughout their careers.

BEST PRACTICE

INSTITUTE PATIENT ADVISORS INTO THE CALL CENTER TRAINING PROGRAM TO SHARE THEIR INTERACTIONS WITH THE CALL CENTER AND TO HELP STAFF DEVELOP EMPATHY AND OTHER SKILLS TO IMPROVE THEIR PERFORMANCE.

Although there are many areas to be covered in a training program, a session dedicated to empathy is essential. Staff members are handling a multitude of calls back to back; it is very easy to forget who is on the other end of the telephone. Reinforce with staff that every call represents a patient, and one who is often struggling with serious medical problems. Recognizing this and empathizing with the caller can help eliminate the belief that the calls being processed are of a routine nature. Since call centers remove face-to-face patient interactions, consider instituting 'patient advisors' into the training plan. Patient advisors can be introduced in training sessions to provide actual examples of failing to meet performance expectations, lack of empathy, and so forth. Instead of just talking about the importance of the patient related to telephone operations, these patients can provide feedback directly to staff. These patient advisors consist of patients within your practice who are willing and interested in dedicating time for improvement efforts. Often, patients are eager to help the practice and can be a valuable resource in improving empathy among the staff. In addition, framing personal stories and pictures of patients within the call center reinforces the importance of displaying empathy in every telephone interaction.

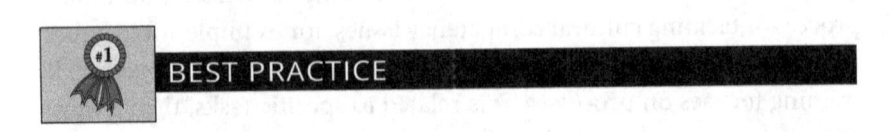

BEST PRACTICE

FRAMING PERSONAL STORIES AND PICTURES OF PATIENTS WITHIN A CALL ENTER REINFORCES THE IMPORTANCE OF DISPLAYING EMPATHY IN EVERY TELEPHONE INTERACTION.

Training initiatives should not just focus on staff within the call center. A practice's successful communication strategy impacts all staff throughout the practice, including providers and nursing staff. Include providers and staff in your development and training processes to identify call hand-off issues or integration opportunities before they negatively affect the performance of the telephone operations.

Career path

A perception exists that the career of a call center employee is limited to answering calls without any real opportunity for growth. Instituting multiple levels of job titles within the call center offers a promotional platform for those staff members that excel. Since call centers often handle more than incoming calls, and incoming calls can vary greatly in complexity, a promotional career path can be a win-win for employee and employer. Exhibit 7.9 provides an example of an approach that offers a three-step promotional path within the call center. This provides growth options for staff, rewards top performers within the center, and can minimize turnover.

Call Center Design

If a call center structure appears to be the right choice for your medical practice, let's cover some key considerations when moving from your practice's current state to the design of the new center.

Focused planning
Spending an appropriate time on the front end of the project by intentionally designing all aspects of the new center pays off with a quicker and less complicated implementation. Always keep the seamless integration of the patient, call center, and medical practice as the beacon of your design process. All decision points need to be compared back to the patient and referring physician experience.

Practice integration
Regardless of the type of call center you decide to build, integration within the practice is critical in delivering high-quality patient care. The call center and the practice must work as a team to resolve the needs of patients and referring physicians. If the call center does not act as the front line for the practice and effectively determine the best avenue for resolution, the practice will be hampered in its ability to deliver high-quality care. If the practice does not respond to the call center, patients are stuck in the middle trying to resolve their own needs. Both must work together in unison for the patient.

To ensure a successful integration, consider developing a "service level agreement" for both parties—the call center and the practice. This agreement should include the quality (for example, abandonment rate, service level and average speed to answer) that is expected to be met or exceeded, the types of calls to be processed by the call center, and the general workflow of messaging as well as live calls. For the practice, the agreement should include a confirmation regarding the general workflow of messages and live calls, as well as the expected response time for live calls that are transferred and messages that are taken.

If a nurse doesn't respond to a message in the timeframe communicated to the patient, for example, the patient will call again only to be greeted by a telephone operator who will have difficulty in managing the now-frustrated caller. Both parties should also agree to the process by which

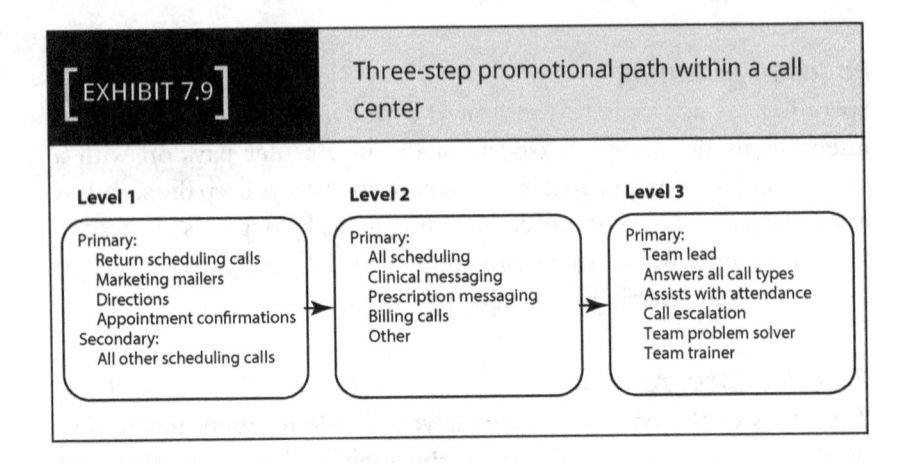

[EXHIBIT 7.9] Three-step promotional path within a call center

Level 1
Primary:
  Return scheduling calls
  Marketing mailers
  Directions
  Appointment confirmations
Secondary:
  All other scheduling calls

Level 2
Primary:
  All scheduling
  Clinical messaging
  Prescription messaging
  Billing calls
  Other

Level 3
Primary:
  Team lead
  Answers all call types
  Assists with attendance
  Call escalation
  Team problem solver
  Team trainer

urgent or emergent calls are escalated, recognizing that the definition of "urgent" and "emergent" are in the hands of the patient or referring physician, not an internal debate between the practice and the call center. By placing workflow and expectations in writing, the practice can avoid challenges regarding the integration of its call center.

Call centers may also benefit from assigning "liaisons" to a practice(s), or rotating staff members at a workstation(s) that is physically located at the practice.

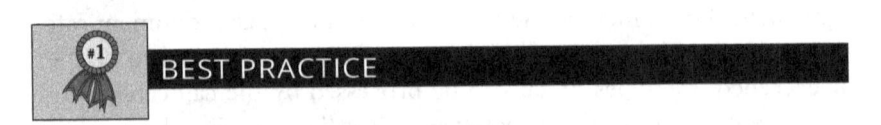

BEST PRACTICE

DEVELOP A SERVICE LEVEL AGREEMENT THAT OUTLINES THE SERVICE EXPECTATIONS OF THE CALL CENTER AND THE PRACTICE. ENSURE THAT THE CALL CENTER MEETS ESTABLISHED QUALITY THRESHOLDS AND THE PRACTICE MEETS CALLBACK TIMELINES.

Call types

A study regarding the types of inbound calls and their volume should be completed before a call center is launched. Outbound calls must also be considered, if applicable. Determine how each type of call will be handled: Will all calls be handled by the call center? Will the call center route calls to another group? Will an ACD be implemented so that certain call types are directly routed to specific groups? Who are the 'groups' who will handle the calls? How will the call center interact with them? Don't just launch a call center to start answering the telephone; develop a detailed process mapping of how all calls will be handled—and who will be held accountable for each stage in the process.

As a part of your study, be sure to measure the number of repeat calls. Repeat calls are not only an indication of inefficiency within the practice, but they will also drive up call center costs. Not only is your call center having to take an additional call, but a repeat call can also double the average handle time as the patient is frustrated and items related to the call must receive immediate attention.

(See Chapter 4 for a detailed discussion regarding measuring telephone calls.)

Vanity number

In order to facilitate easy recognition of the telephone number, practices may choose to maintain a vanity number. This term is used to describe a telephone number that can be easily recalled by a patient, family member, referring physician or any other caller. Often a toll-free number, the numbers—or associated letters—are placed in a sequence so as to ensure they are easily remembered. The vanity number may be a series of numbers—for example, 888-888-1234—or a term associated with the practice or a specific service—for example, 877-4-HEALTH or 231-MY-BONES. These numbers are derived with input from marketing experts, either internal resources or via a vendor.

While a vanity number may seem to be the first action step of a call center, it's important to be aware that anyone can call the vanity number for any reason. Thus, the practice cannot simply route all of these calls to a scheduler trained to handle a specific physician or service. A vanity number requires an operator(s), and a well-defined workflow to ensure that the operator(s) can reach or transfer the caller to someone who can handle their call. Training is also required to address the multitude of calls that represent general inquiries about your practice. This may include your location, physicians, services, and so forth. A vanity number invites "curious" callers. Of course, the goal is to convert those callers into patients, however, it requires skill and access to resources.

Because of this dynamic, it is common to see a call center start with its 'legacy' number(s), and subsequently build the infrastructure needed for a vanity number.

Location

The location of the call center influences the level of attention that is paid to maintaining a cohesive team within the practice. If a call center is located off-site (which could mean across the street), the battle to avoid the "us against them" mentality must begin immediately. Similarly, if the call center has a remote employee program, with staff working from their homes, it is important to make efforts to connect these employees to the clinical practice. Off-site call centers need a plan that includes periodic face-to-face meetings between call center staff and the team at the practice. Attempt to conduct meetings outside of business hours so that call center employees can attend and be involved in the team. These meetings should occur at least quarterly to foster continued communication. Ensure that an agenda item within each meeting specifically addresses the call center/practice integration and communication. If you can't conduct after-hours meetings that everyone can attend, identify a rotating staff member who is assigned to attend meetings at the practice and be the representative for the call center. It is his or her responsibility to share call-center-related items with practice staff and also disseminate information back at the call center. Using a protocol to rotate the call center representative allows everyone the opportunity to integrate with the practice.

If open dialogue from the practice is not well planned, scheduling errors and other such miscommunications can inundate the call center and prevent it from focusing on performance improvement initiatives. When providers perceive that a call center employee cannot accurately schedule their patients, for example, mistrust ensues. To foster open communication, develop and promote the use of a simple form to facilitate feedback from providers and staff. The feedback form, preferably electronic, should be formulated in a manner such that a physician, provider, nurse, or other staff member can quickly complete and transmit it to the call center. The form should include the patient's name, date of birth, and any other qualifiers needed to identify the patient along with the error (reported by the caller or perceived to have occurred). When feedback is received, the call center must have an established process to research and provide timely resolution back to the physician, provider, nurse, or other staff member with any action steps taken. The ability to pull recorded calls and investigate the conversation, as discussed previously, is paramount in determining the cause of the complaint. Otherwise, call centers will always be managing within a "he said/she said" environment.

Once researched, provide a timely response and be specific about the cause of the complaint. If the problem was a scheduling error on the staff member's part, for example, provide specifics about what actions will be taken to ensure that this does not happen again.

Stakeholders

Migrating the operations of the primary communication vehicle in a practice—the telephones—results in changes for all stakeholders.

In addition to the changes that patients and referring physicians will experience, internal stakeholders—to include staff, practice administration, and providers—will undergo change. Treat the conversion to a new communication model as an opportunity for improvement, not as a detriment. During the transition from a model consisting of decentralized telephone operations to one that features a call center model, timely communication to all parties involved is crucial.

Every stakeholder has a different opinion, and effort must be taken to manage their perceptions while the reality is being altered. Displaying a constant effort toward process improvement and transparency enables the practice to build the trust of stakeholders.

- **Staff.** If your practice pursues the development of a call center, make sure employees know what to expect, as they will be concerned not only about the changes involved in the transition, but also the prospect of job losses. Involve an optimistic employee who has the respect of his or her peers in the design process of the call center. Publicly acknowledge the staff member and commend the employee for his or her effort and insightful vision. This recognition keeps the team member on task and motivated. If another successful call center is located in close proximity to your practice, plan a site visit for your staff. Even if the call center is not in the healthcare industry, the visit aids management and employees in understanding the call center initiative. (Indeed, visiting a call center outside of the industry is a great idea to really engage staff in performance improvement; they see new ideas and methods that can be imported.) A site visit can demonstrate how a well operated call center can be successful for all parties.

- **Administration.** It is not uncommon for practice leaders to carry a negative connotation because of personal experiences or anecdotes from other poorly executed call centers. It is important for the administration to recognize and embrace the benefits of a call center for the practice and, most importantly, the patients' experience. Practice leaders must publicly support the transition with physicians, providers, nurses, staff, and referring physicians' offices. Moreover, they must be able to articulate the vision of the call center. The administration must help set realistic expectations; it is typical to experience a slight degrading of performance during the transition. New processes need to be ironed out, and staff requires time to adjust to the new protocols and associated expectations. Ensure that all stakeholders understand that some pitfalls are expected in the transition so you can work to resolve any issues instead of concentrating on damage control with leadership.

- **Clinicians.** Physicians and other clinicians, as well as their clinical staff, might have numerous reasons why they believe a call center will not work. Including clinicians throughout the decision and design process is vital. Develop a timely, comprehensive communication plan for providers to ensure that they understand what the practice is trying to achieve. Include illustrations regarding the expected return on investment in terms of patient and referring physician satisfaction, increased appointments, and reduced abandonment rates. Recognize that the most common pushback from clinicians is: "my practice is too complex for a call center to manage."

Don't just start by employing new staff to answer and handle calls. Prior to implementing a call center, review and understand operations and workflow of the practice, to include the scheduling protocols of all physicians and providers. If current scheduling protocols require a doctorate to schedule the patient accurately, then effort must be made to simplify and streamline schedules, and standardize protocols. The knowledge database discussed previously is a great tool to foster embedding protocols in the scheduling process to ensure accuracy.

Perhaps the best information to present is feedback from patients and referring physicians who—if the practice takes the time to listen—are likely to share frustration regarding accessing the practice via its current telephone system. Instill in all stakeholders that a successful call center is an investment, not a cost. When effectively operated, a call center is an essential driver of profits throughout the practice.

> **BEST PRACTICE**
>
> A SUCCESSFUL CALL CENTER IS AN INVESTMENT, NOT A COST. WHEN EFFECTIVELY OPERATED, A CALL CENTER IS AN ESSENTIAL DRIVER OF PRACTICE PROFITS.

Summary

A call center can be an effective model to improve the communications of a practice, as well as patient access and service. To determine if your practice will benefit from a call center, evaluate your current telephone access and determine the magnitude of improvement opportunity. If a call center is implemented, be diligent in its design, staffing, and communication protocols.

CHAPTER 8

Virtual Communication and Telehealth

The telephone, in its exclusive use for voice-to-voice exchange, is becoming a legacy system. Increasingly, telephones, or their more popular name as "smartphones," are being used for text and electronic communication. In the future, patients will neither be encouraged nor required to use the telephone to communicate with a medical practice. Technologies such as patient portals, virtual visits, web chat and social media are coming to the forefront as a means for patients to engage with their medical practice.

For the foreseeable future, however, the telephone will continue to remain a critical pipeline for patients, referring physicians, hospitals, nursing homes, pharmacies, and other stakeholders to communicate with the medical practice. At the same time, medical practices need to transition to provide options for patient engagement that do not rely on the telephone. Virtual communication and telehealth represent a value proposition for both patients and practices.

Patients need access to care 24 hours a day, seven days a week, not simply during standard business office hours. Patients want to have their concerns addressed when and where they need it. Virtual communication and telehealth represent a disruptive innovation in the healthcare delivery system brought about via a combination of the following:

Virtual Technology: We are busy sending texts, chats, and images over the telephone via our thumbs, not conducting a high volume of verbal, synchronous exchanges between caller and receiver. Technology exists today to hold patient-facing visits via web-based video services; and physicians can communicate with one other via e-consults by sharing data, images and medical records to obtain consults without the need for a patient-facing visit. And the technology exists today for patients to integrate health and wellness in each aspect of their lives, via mobile health devices and remote care.

Immediacy to Care: Patients are now financially engaged in their care via high deductibles, copayments and co-insurance and they are seeking immediate care and answers. The value for their healthcare dollar is based not only on the quality of care they receive, but also on access to care. Having to place a telephone call to the medical practice, wait on hold and be given an appointment days or weeks later is simply not how countless people live their lives. Many do not understand why they cannot obtain care and information when and where they need it. The rise in mobile health devices have met some of the demand for immediate information. Wearable digital devices and remote biometric monitoring have been integrated into many patients' lives, offering instantaneous feedback. Yet, practices have many opportunities to provide immediacy to care.

Provider Shortages: The shortages of clinicians have led to disruptive innovation in the healthcare industry. A specialty physician can provide e-consults to community physicians in real time, thereby collapsing the time to care while also increasing provider efficiency. With community and family members serving as an extended healthcare workforce, the eyes and ears for the clinical care team have expanded. Non-healthcare workers are now conducting remote monitoring of vital signs in the home (or office) and ensuring medication is taken as prescribed. Care teams are relying on family and community to ensure population health and wellness.

Transitions of Care: The recognition that the hand-offs of care between one provider and the next or one facility and the next are a vital step in improving health outcomes has led to advances in the use of telehealth with patients and caregivers. Transitional care management is one of the new frontiers of healthcare. Efforts have gone well beyond simply calling patients via telephone soon after discharge. It involves a timely interaction to plan for the next transition, electronically communicating the information, equipment and supplies needed so the next step in the patient's care can become seamless, thereby extending the care continuum of the patient.

Reimbursement Reform: More and more, insurers and employers are recognizing the advantages of immediate access to care. They are changing their reimbursement methods accordingly. The federal government has also recognized the importance of transitional care management, chronic care management and virtual access, with new CPT codes. Slowly, but surely, the transition to population health management is taking place in the financing of healthcare.

These change catalysts have led many healthcare organizations to alter their delivery systems to align with new, automated care delivery and communication platforms. Telehealth is a broad term that refers to obtaining healthcare services and/or healthcare information electronically. Consider expanding your practice's telehealth capabilities.

Patient Portal

The patient portal was first introduced as a central point of contact for patients to obtain information about their health. Patients were encouraged to acquire log-in information to securely access their test results, request an appointment, request a medication renewal, pay their bill and other similar clinical and business access.

Take the following steps to expand the functionality and usage of your patient portal:

First, determine the extent to which your current portal is being used. Although you can commence with understanding how many patients have registered with your portal, the key is usage. What percentage of your patients utilize the portal and with what frequency? What are the reasons they are using the portal?

Second, examine the reasons for your inbound telephone call demand. Determine what types of telephone calls can be reduced if additional services are available to patients via your portal.

In better performing practices, the patient portal is expanded to provide an interactive dialogue between the patient and the care team in the form of secure messaging, as well as to permit patients to actively contribute to their health record as part of a healthcare partnership with their care team. The challenge for many of today's medical practices is the right balance of clinical staff to manage telephones and portal messages, achieved via first-call or first-touch resolution.

BEST PRACTICE

EXPAND YOUR PATIENT PORTAL TO PROVIDE AN INTERACTIVE DIALOGUE BETWEEN THE PATIENT AND THE CARE TEAM IN THE FORM OF SECURE MESSAGING AND PERMIT PATIENTS TO ACTIVELY CONTRIBUTE TO THEIR HEALTH RECORD AS PART OF A HEALTHCARE PARTNERSHIP WITH THEIR CARE TEAM.

Virtual Visits

Virtual visits refer to patient visits that occur outside of the traditional office visit setting. These may include televisits, whereby the patient and caregiver are synchronously on the telephone having a conversation, as well as newer methods of electronic patient-facing visits to include a secure, web-based video interchange. Some of these visits also combine interactive data, such as remote monitoring and digital photos. Recognizing specialty shortages in many markets, a virtual visit can be highly beneficial to communities in need of your specialty expertise. Telehealth services provide access to care that may otherwise be unavailable and can extend the reach of your practice.

Is it time for your practice to begin to offer virtual visits? If so, investigate the following for your practice:

BEST PRACTICE

VIRTUAL VISITS REFER TO PATIENT-FACING VISITS THAT OCCUR OUTSIDE OF THE TRADITIONAL OFFICE VISIT SETTING. INVESTIGATE YOUR VISIT TYPES, WAIT TIME TO APPOINTMENT, AND AFTER-HOURS CARE TO DETERMINE IF IT IS TIME FOR YOUR PRACTICE TO BEGIN TO OFFER VIRTUAL VISITS.

Visit types: Examine your face-to-face visits and determine whether each of the visits need to be conducted in the office setting, face-to-face with the provider. As an example, is a face-to-face visit to the urologist needed if the patient has been diagnosed with kidney stones? What type of data is learned in the face-to-face visit and can that information be learned via other means? As another example, for a screening colonoscopy on a patient without symptoms or family history, is a pre-procedure face-to-face visit needed or can the pertinent patient history be taken via other means?

Wait time to appointment: What is the wait time to appointment for your physicians? If your wait time today is similar to what it was three weeks ago, recognize that your practice is in a constant state. You will likely continue to have these wait times for the foreseeable future until you take action. Which visits could be expedited by having a virtual visit with the patient, thereby reducing or collapsing the wait time to appointment? Can some patients receive asynchronous encounters via secure messaging, such as patients with chronic disease?

After hours care: Where are your patients seeking and receiving care after hours? If your practice is a patient-centered medical home or otherwise held accountable for value-based care, is a newer delivery system needed to meet patient needs on a 24/7 basis? If so, explore the utilization and feasibility of round-the-clock nurse triage and advice with scheduling capability and same-day access capability (such as walk-in clinics, urgent care clinics, provider-of-the-day, or advanced access scheduling). What is the return-on-investment of these access methods versus a telehealth or video visit with patients?

If the decision is made to pursue virtual visits, ask and answer the following questions.

Technology: What technology is needed in the practice to carry out a secure televisit or video visit with the patient? What are the requirements for back-up? Will the visit be permanently recorded or translated to a note in the chart? What security is needed related to the technology to ensure compliance with HIPAA and other regulations?

Provider 'credit': How will providers be credited with this work? As an example, should this work volume be tracked and formally recognized as part of the measurement, if applicable, of provider production, e.g., via assigned wRVUs or other methods?

Reimbursement: Is there an opportunity to submit bills to insurers for telehealth, and be paid as a covered service? If so, what are the requirements to bill and collect for these services?

E-consults

Many of the large healthcare delivery systems have extended their reach by offering physician-to-physician telehealth. In these systems, a specialist is available via e-consult to another provider in 'real time' as they are seeing their patient, or within 24 to 48 hours after the patient's visit. The ability to offer e-consults collapses the time to care for patients, as they no longer need to wait for the referral process to occur to learn the next step in their care. Instead, an e-consult occurs between providers so that the appropriate next step in the patient's care can be secured earlier in the process. This may include the need to order a test or image, expedite treatment or intervention based on the patient's status, provide remote education to providers and/or patients and other means. In this fashion, the limited resource of the specialist is extended and the specialist's time is efficiently spent on seeing those patients that truly require a face-to-face visit. Primary care physicians benefit from timely access to specialty expertise—and the reassurance that their patient is being appropriately serviced to ensure the highest quality of care.

> **BEST PRACTICE**
>
> ARE E-CONSULTS IN YOUR FUTURE? THE ABILITY TO OFFER E-CONSULTS COLLAPSES THE TIME TO CARE FOR PATIENTS, AS THEY NO LONGER NEED TO WAIT FOR THE REFERRAL PROCESS TO OCCUR TO LEARN THE NEXT STEP IN THEIR CARE. IDENTIFY THE TECHNOLOGY PLATFORM NEEDED TO FACILITATE THIS OPPORTUNITY AS YOU INTEGRATE THIS IN YOUR TELEHEALTH PROGRAM.

Are e-consults in your future? Determine the types of referrals you are receiving today. Are some of them inappropriate or could be better managed by another practice or specialist? If so, develop education materials for your referring physicians, such as a referral checklist, to ensure that the prerequisite tests, data and interventions have been taken prior to referral. Consider whether an e-consult between physicians will provide for improved care transition. Most importantly, identify the technology platform needed to facilitate this opportunity as you integrate this in your telehealth program.

Summary

In summary, evaluate whether it is time to grow your e-access clinical and business capabilities. Interactive, real-time access to information and care fully integrates healthcare into a patient's daily life.

CHAPTER 9

Communication Tools

What the caller hears and how you present yourself on the telephone define the caller's impression of your practice's access. Experts agree, customers develop their impression of a business within the first 10 seconds, and that's just about the length of time it takes to greet a caller on the telephone. It's your opportunity to make it a great impression, and you can accomplish that with telephone scripts, quality communication, and tools to support your efforts.

In this chapter, we discuss tools and resources to execute successful telephone access to your practice:

- Telephone scripts to help ensure consistent, high-quality telephone interactions;
- Tools to enhance nonverbal communication;
- Customer service tools to improve service access and delivery; and
- Telephone message tools to ensure accurate and complete messages.

BEST PRACTICE

PRINT RIBBONS TO HANG UNDER YOUR NAMETAGS OR SMALL SIGNS TO ADHERE TO YOUR WORKSTATIONS THAT SAY "THE FIRST 10 SECONDS." THIS MESSAGE SERVES AS A REMINDER OF THE IMPORTANCE OF YOUR INITIAL INTERACTION WITH THE CALLER.

Telephone Scripts

Use standard telephone scripts to ensure a consistent experience for callers. There are two methods of scripting: (1) design the specific words to say and (2) provide an outline of key information. For a telephone call greeting and closure, which are consistently used in each call, highlight the specific words for staff to say to callers. Given the nature of a medical practice (and the hundreds of reasons that a caller is communicating with you), it's nearly impossible to provide specific scripts for staff to follow for each type of call. Instead, an effective management tool is to provide outlines based on call type of the practice's expectations for the information that should be gathered and/or communicated during the call. As an example, Exhibit 9.1 presents a list of information that should be outlined for appointment-related calls.

Although the reasons for calls vary, develop written protocols for handling frequent situations, such as those presented in Exhibit 9.2. Give staff members the tools they need to effectively manage each

[EXHIBIT 9.1] Information to be scripted for appointment calls

- Scripted greeting (see 'The greeting' section on p. 173);
- Appointment information (provider, day of week, date, time, and location); repeat this information to the patient at the conclusion of the call;
- Request to complete and submit registration and medical history online, as applicable, while revealing—and repeating—the practice's website or patient portal;
- Reminder to bring proper identification, insurance card(s), payment, and referral information;
- Statement of account balance, as applicable, with an offer to accept a credit/debit card payment from the patient if willing and able;
- Preparation instructions for any tests, as applicable;
- Directions (patients may be directed to website or transferred to an extension that provides automated directions); and
- Scripted closure (see 'The closing' section on p. 174).

> **[EXHIBIT 9.2] Develop scripts for frequent scenarios**
>
> - Does not speak English
> - Is having a medical emergency
> - Has the wrong number
> - Has a clinical question
> - Requests a prescription
> - Asks to speak with a physician or staff member
> - Asks to have results of a test
> - Wants to update his or her personal or insurance information
> - Wants a copy of his or her medical record
> - Wants to discuss his or her bill
> - Has a complaint
> - Asks personal questions regarding patients (for example, father calls to see if his son is a patient of your practice)

caller (the same scripts/tools also apply to portal and text based patient communications).

As Exhibit 9.2 demonstrates, many common questions are asked each day; script responses to enable the operator to get right to the point. Directions to the office or referred testing sites, as well as the name of the provider on call, should always be handy. Reinforce the importance of using telephone scripts by incorporating compliance with scripting in your staff performance management process. Provide staff members with the telephone scripts they need to manage the telephones and then hold them accountable for using these important tools.

BEST PRACTICE

SAMPLE SCRIPT: "I WOULD BE HAPPY TO ANSWER YOUR QUESTION, AND YOU MAY FIND OTHER USEFUL INFORMATION ON OUR WEBSITE [OR PORTAL] AT WWW.PRACTICENAME.COM."

In addition to scripting common telephone scenarios, train staff to recognize situations in which calls need to be escalated and emergencies. Give staff the guidelines to handle extenuating circumstances with referring physicians. Be sure to provide this training to staff members who you believe would never even answer your telephones—even the lab technician who might pick up a call now and then. We're not suggesting that the lab technician step into the role of your triage nurse, but you never know who will be around when a crisis occurs. An informed staff contributes to ensuring an efficient practice. Preparation is good risk management and patient service.

BEST PRACTICE

POST ANSWERS TO COMMON QUESTIONS ON YOUR PRACTICE'S WEBSITE OR PATIENT PORTAL, THEREBY REDUCING THE NEED FOR PATIENTS TO CALL YOU WITH ROUTINE QUESTIONS.

If you can anticipate some of the callers' questions, post them with the correct responses on your practice's website or portal in a "Frequently Asked Questions" section. This may reduce the volume of calls from patients asking routine questions. Whenever appropriate, direct callers to information provided on your practice's website, patient portal, or via the patient's personal health record. Although it may take one or two verbal reminders, callers will slowly but surely get in the habit of checking for information online (or wherever you may direct them) instead of calling. Avoiding the need for a call—while still meeting the caller's expectations—is a strategy that promotes the goals of providing consistently good patient service. (See Chapter 5 for more ideas on alternatives to calls.)

[CHAPTER 9] | COMMUNICATION TOOLS

BEST PRACTICE

KEEP WRITING TABLETS NEAR ALL TELEPHONES. AS SOON AS THE CALLER STATES HIS OR HER NAME, WRITE IT DOWN. OTHERWISE, YOU MAY FORGET THE NAME AS YOU LISTEN TO THE DETAILS OF THE REQUEST, FORCING YOU TO ASK FOR THE CALLER'S NAME AGAIN AS THE CONVERSATION ENSUES. THE CALLER MAY WONDER WHAT OTHER INFORMATION YOU MISSED. AFTER YOU HAVE THE NAME, USE IT AS OFTEN AS YOU CAN DURING THE CONVERSATION. THE NAME OFFERS A CONNECTION TO THE PATIENT AND DEMONSTRATES THAT YOU ARE LISTENING AND ATTENTIVE. CAPTURING IT AT THE BEGINNING ALSO ALLOWS THE STAFF MEMBER TO QUERY THE PATIENT'S ACCOUNT TO EFFECTIVELY TAKE A MESSAGE VIA THE EHR SYSTEM.

The greeting

Each caller should have a consistently positive experience when telephoning your practice. To ensure uniform and reliable experience for callers, we recommend four elements in the greeting:

1. Welcome: Acknowledge and welcome the caller. Example: "Good morning."
2. Identification: State the name of the practice and/or department.
3. Operator's first name.
4. Query Example: "How may I help you?"

Incorporating these four elements into each greeting is a small but important step that ensures each caller gets a consistently high level of service.

In the greeting, use the full name of your practice, avoiding any slang ("Ped-e-G-I," for example, for a pediatric gastroenterology practice). It may be quicker for your receptionist to say, "Hello, Surg Onc" (as opposed to "Hello, Surgical Oncology Associates"), but you'll lose time in the long run as callers pause and wonder if they've reached the right place. Everyone who answers a telephone should say your practice's name with as few abbreviations as possible. It makes a more professional impression and ultimately contributes to a higher level of service. Remember that this initial greeting is a distinct marketing opportunity to state your brand to every caller, so use the opportunity to express it appropriately and consistently.

For example: "Good morning. You have reached Medical Practice Associates. This is Sally speaking. How may I help you?" This should be a routine part of how each telephone call is answered.

The closing

In addition to a consistent greeting, conclude each call with a standard closure. Instruct staff to use the caller's name—"Ms. Jones" or "Mr. Smith," for example—at the end of conversations. Indeed, feel free to use the caller's name several times during the conversation. Stating the patient's name reinforces the fact that you are actively listening.

Go a step further and thank patients for choosing your practice, particularly when scheduling an appointment. Conclude calls by asking callers if there is anything else they need. For example: "Thank you for choosing Medical Practice Associates for your care, Ms. Jones. Is there anything else I can do to help you?" If performed consistently, you'll leave a positive and memorable impression.

BEST PRACTICE

CONCLUDE EVERY CALL WITH "THANK YOU FOR CHOOSING OUR PRACTICE FOR YOUR CARE." IT DEMONSTRATES YOUR APPRECIATION—AND ACKNOWLEDGES THE FACT THAT THE PATIENT MADE A CHOICE.

[EXHIBIT 9.3] Positive response sets

When you cannot provide the caller's desired outcome—there are no earlier openings on the appointment schedule, for example—shift the language from a negative to a positive by informing callers what you can do (vs. what you can't do).

Instead of saying:	"No. I can't help you."
Respond this way:	When a patient calls late in the day with a nonurgent medical question, for example, but the clinical staff has already left the office, reply by saying: "The office staff has left for the day, but they will be in tomorrow morning at 9 a.m., and I will have the nurse contact you at that time. Is the 555.555.5555 number a good one to use or is there a better number to reach you tomorrow?"
Instead of saying:	"Hang on a second."
Respond this way:	"It may take me a few minutes to research this. Are you able to hold while I check or shall I take your number to call you back?"
Instead of saying:	"You'll have to …"
Respond this way:	Give a response that does not appear to tell the patient what he or she has to do. Instead, reply by saying: "Here's how we can help you with that…. Is this acceptable?"
Instead of saying:	"Dr. _____ is not in the office today."
Respond this way:	"Dr. _____ is not in the office today. How may I help you?"
Instead of saying:	"She's at lunch."
Respond this way:	"I am sorry, but she is not available. May I have her call you later or may I be of assistance?"
Instead of:	Ignoring the patient's comments;
Respond this way:	"I am sorry that you are not feeling well," or a similar remark, to acknowledge the patient's comment and, in the event that the patient is upset, to diffuse the situation.

Positive response sets

Although scripts cannot be written for each possible scenario, staff members can be educated to use particular words and phrases. The words they choose when responding to callers should reflect a positive response set rather than a negative one. Scripts also help educate staff to enhanced verbal communication skills. As a service industry, patients do not want to be treated as a number or a disease. Instead, professional, compassionate, and service-oriented behaviors can be taught through repetitive scripting and customer-minded tools.

Review the examples in Exhibit 9.3 with staff while asking for feedback about other positive responses to use—or negative ones to avoid.

BEST PRACTICE

THE TELEPHONE CAN LEAVE STAFF MEMBERS WITH THE IMPRESSION THAT THEY ARE SOMEHOW DETACHED FROM PATIENT CARE. EMPHASIZE THAT EVERY TELEPHONE CALL IS A LIFE. PARTICULARLY FOR TELEPHONE STAFF WHO ARE NOT LOCATED IN THE CLINICAL AREA, HANG PICTURES OF PATIENTS AS A REMINDER OF THE IMPORTANT CONNECTION THAT TELEPHONE STAFF MEMBERS HAVE WITH PATIENTS EVEN WHEN THEY CAN'T SEE THEM FACE TO FACE.

Information requests

Make sure your employees have the requisite knowledge to answer common questions posed by callers. We have witnessed numerous instances where employees have not been given the information to respond to callers. The questions in Exhibit 9.4 reflect the sophistication

[EXHIBIT 9.4] Patient inquiries that require expanded knowledge

- Which one of the physicians would you select for your own healthcare (or your child's)?
- Where did the physician train?
- How many _____ procedures does he (or she) do each year?
- What is his (or her) complication rate for this procedure?
- How much will the procedure cost?

of today's patients—and the lack of training for many telephone staff members to respond to specific questions regarding the medical practice. Ask your employees to jot down the questions they receive and create standard information protocols for staff to use when responding to patients. Large practices often integrate this information into knowledge databases that are integrated in their practice management system—or on a separate electronic platform that is readily accessible by staff members.

Staff Knowledge

Patients pose many clinical questions when they call your medical practice. To gauge the quality of telephone contact with patients, many practices ask the question: "Is the staff knowledgeable?" as part of their patient satisfaction survey. Although most clinical staff members regard themselves as very informed, educated, and conversant, some patients don't come to that conclusion, particularly during telephone conversations. When a patient asks a question about his or her treatment or test results, it's common for a clinical staff member to respond: "Let me ask Dr. Smith."

It's no surprise that patients are concerned about this staff member's knowledge—he or she never gives information without checking first with the physician. Patients do not differentiate whether the staff member is reluctant to release information without the physician's approval—or just doesn't know the answer. Patients tend to assume it is the latter. Adding to the mix are the frustrations involved with the delays that some patients experience waiting for a return call.

To improve the process, sit down and determine patients' most frequently asked questions. Ask your physicians if they are willing to develop new guidelines or clinical protocols, in writing, that permit clinical staff to respond to some of the patients' inquiries, while also clarifying when the physician should become involved in the issue. For example, basic postoperative wound care could be included in the new guidelines, with the clinical staff providing this education to patients and responding to patients' inquiries regarding their care. So, too, clear guidance should be developed about which questions should be referred to the physician immediately versus those that can be responded to later in the day.

In addition to the new guidelines, it's important for clinical staff members to change their responses to patients' questions that truly do need the physician's response. In these situations, train the nurses and medical assistants to respond: "That is a very important question, and I know that Dr. Smith would like to hear it. I'd like to run it by her and get back to you." This new response positions the clinical staff as an integral member of the care team. The old way of responding ("Let me ask Dr. Smith") works to perpetuate a reliance on the physician to personally manage all calls rather than engender confidence in the clinical care team.

If your physicians are willing and your clinical team is up to the challenge, these changes in workflow related to telephone calls can improve patient communication and practice efficiency.

Nonverbal Communication Tools

Simply managing the inbound telephone call by imparting consistent information is not sufficient. In fact, we've all had interactions with a person over the telephone where we knew that the information we received was accurate and comprehensive, but the manner in which we received it was totally inappropriate. In groundbreaking research, UCLA Professor Emeritus Albert Mehrabian concluded that only 18 percent of a customer's experience was related to the words used, while an overwhelmingly 82 percent of the caller's experience was defined by the vocal qualities of the operator (see Exhibit 9.5).

By studying and improving your vocal quality, staff can improve each caller's experience with your practice. Ensure that callers feel they are being treated with respect, courtesy, and compassion by focusing on a positive display of the following vocal qualities:

- Tone: Expression of feeling or emotion
- Rate: Number of words spoken per minute
- Inflection: Emphasizing words and syllables to enhance the verbal encounter
- Pitch: Highness or deepness of voice
- Volume: How loud or soft the voice sounds

Train staff to retain the information about these characteristics by remembering the acronym 'TRIPV.'

One of the key vocal qualities, the rate of speaking, can convey 'urgency' to a voice as if the operator needs to hurry callers along so they can get to the next caller. This is easily perceived by callers as a lack of interest and 'coldness' rather than compassion and caring. It's true that some callers may have a hard time getting to the point. Instead of speaking at a rapid rate, help them along by politely asking, "What may I help you with,

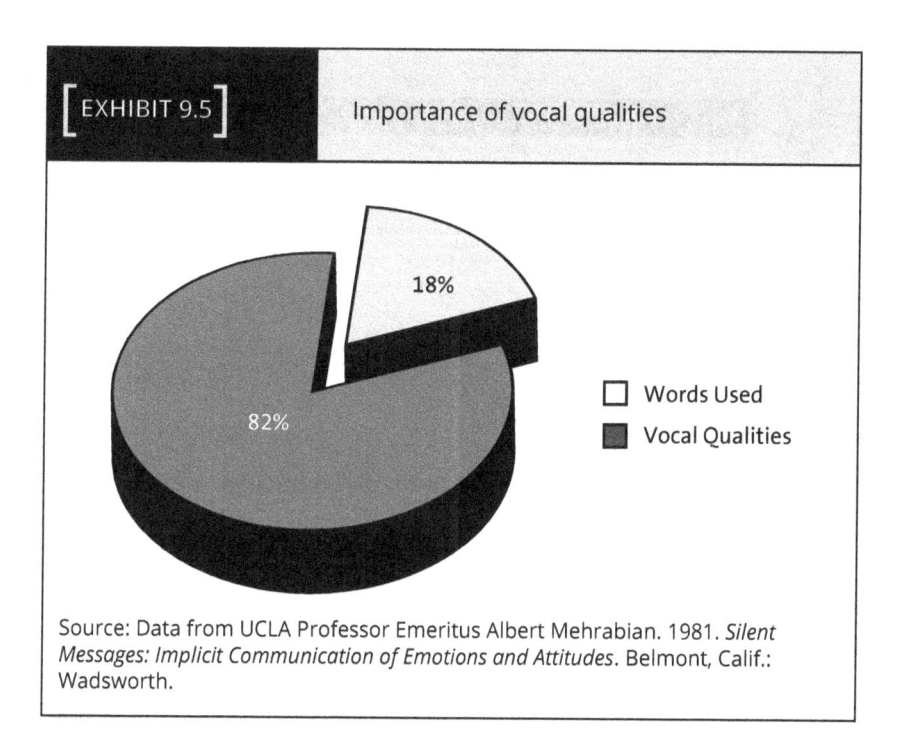

[EXHIBIT 9.5] Importance of vocal qualities

- 18% Words Used
- 82% Vocal Qualities

Source: Data from UCLA Professor Emeritus Albert Mehrabian. 1981. *Silent Messages: Implicit Communication of Emotions and Attitudes*. Belmont, Calif.: Wadsworth.

Ms. Jones?" during a pause (or even a breath) in their statement. Try role playing during a staff meeting to show staff how to help patients get to the point without being perceived as pushy.

Ask your staff members about examples of positive—and negative—vocal qualities that they have personally experienced. Using these scenarios, as well as ones from your practice, role-play the required tone, rate, inflection, pitch, and volume that you expect of staff.

A bad mood or lousy attitude seems to leap through the telephone. Watch for inadvertent nonverbal communication, such as sighs or moans. Beware of talking too rapidly or loudly as well as using a condescending or inappropriate tone. You can sense someone's attitude through the telephone. Make a point of smiling as you speak—patients will sense that smile—even over the telephone. Try putting a mirror on the wall in front of telephone staff members and ask them to smile sincerely when they answer each call, just as they would be expected to in a face-to-face encounter.

BEST PRACTICE

YOU CAN SENSE SOMEONE'S ATTITUDE THROUGH THE TELEPHONE. MAKE A POINT OF SMILING AS YOU SPEAK—PATIENTS WILL SENSE THAT SMILE—EVEN OVER THE TELEPHONE.

Customer Service Tools

Beyond the professionalism, courtesy, and empathy perceived by patients when they contact your medical practice, a number of customer service tools can help when interactions with the patient do not go as planned.

These difficult "moments of truth" are often the benchmark that patients use to assess your medical practice's quality. Indeed, for many patients, their assessment of your service serves as a proxy for their perception of your quality. Many patients may not have the knowledge and tools to assess clinical quality, but they certainly have the knowledge and tools to assess your level of service.

Keep your service promise

Make sure staff members understand the importance of keeping their service promise. If the patient is informed that he or she will receive a return call—referred to as a "callback"—in three hours, place the call to the patient in three hours (or respond to a portal message)—even if it means that the patient will only be informed of an update rather than a resolution to his or her inquiry. Keeping your service promise reflects on your practice's integrity and influences the confidence patients have in your practice. Plus, it vastly reduces the work associated with repeat calls.

Practice service recovery

A medical practice is a service organization. Although we hope that every interaction with the patient is positive, some fall short of our expectations. When this occurs, be sure to have a ready response that is fair and equitable to all callers who experience a problem situation. For example, order a small bouquet of flowers to be delivered to a patient to apologize for the fact they were lost on hold for two hours, or send them a small gift card or a written note of apology. Be sure you do not become extravagant or your gift may be construed as an inducement for referrals to your practice. See Exhibit 9.6 for an advisory opinion from the Office of the Inspector General. Work with your legal counsel and malpractice carrier regarding service recovery that is appropriate for the situation.

Manage complaints

Perhaps the most important response to learn is reacting to a caller's complaint. Instead of being defensive (easy to feel that way because the complaint received by the telephone operator is typically about an issue over which the operator has no control), reply with a positive statement.

> **[EXHIBIT 9.6]   Remuneration for service failures**
>
> A health system requested guidance from the Office of the Inspector General (OIG) regarding the use of gift cards for service failures. The cards are $10 in value, with a limit of $50 per annum, redeemable at certain local vendors, excluding the health system. The program would not be advertised. Historically, the OIG has considered any remuneration to patient as an inducement for referrals. On July 28, 2008, the OIG issued a statement in favor of the gift cards: "we conclude that (i) the Proposed Arrangement would not constitute prohibited remuneration within the meaning of section 1128A(a)(5) of the Act; and (ii) while the Proposed Arrangement could potentially generate prohibited remuneration under the anti-kickback statute, if the requisite intent to induce or reward referrals of Federal healthcare program business were present, the OIG would not impose administrative sanctions ..."
>
> Source: OIG Advisory Opinion No. 08-07.

When a patient complains, make an affirmative statement; for example: "Thank you for bringing that to our attention" or "I'm sorry that we didn't meet your expectations." These statements often diffuse caller frustration, as the caller feels recognized and appreciated.

BEST PRACTICE

> WHEN A CALLER COMPLAINS, MAKE AN AFFIRMATIVE STATEMENT SUCH AS "THANK YOU FOR BRINGING THAT TO OUR ATTENTION" OR "I'M SORRY THAT WE DIDN'T MEET YOUR EXPECTATIONS." THE MANAGER SHOULD CALL EVERY PATIENT WHO REGISTERS A FORMAL COMPLAINT. EVEN IF THE COMPLAINT CANNOT BE RESOLVED, THE ACKNOWLEDGMENT ALONE PROVES TO THE PATIENT THAT THE PRACTICE RECOGNIZES ITS PATIENTS' CONCERNS.

Use the patient's name in the conversation; it demonstrates that you are listening. Write down the caller's comments to verbally summarize at the conclusion of the conversation; it indicates that you took the complaint seriously. Many callers just want to be heard. If possible, state the next step that you will take with the complaint; such as giving a note to the physician or nurse. For patients who want an answer to their complaint, give realistic expectations about response times.

If the caller has a complaint about your practice or is simply taking out their bad mood on you, don't absorb their emotions. Help staff resist the urge to respond negatively. Post a quote, photo, or some other calming focal point at staff workstations. It will give them something to focus on when difficult situations arise. Provide a script that is easy for the staff to remember, such as "thank you for bringing that to our attention, Ms. Jones."

Also, give staff a process for escalating the call to a manager and the scripting to permit this smooth transition of a disgruntled caller. For example, consider the following script: "Thank you for bringing this to our attention. I want to be sure my manager has an opportunity to talk with you directly about this issue. Are you able to hold for two minutes while I locate her or can I have her call you back within the next 30 minutes?" This works to diffuse some of the caller's emotion by signifying to the caller the importance of the issue or complaint but also buys some time to allow the caller to calm down. After the manager has called the patient to review the complaint, he or she should record the patient's name, date, time, and issue for the practice's leadership to review. Incorporating complaints about the telephone (and other issues) in a log or spreadsheet on a shared drive accessible by all staff members provides a basis to discover and address the root causes of complaints and to understand the roles the practice's staff, processes, or equipment may play in creating or failing to sufficiently resolve the situation. The manager should call every patient who registers a formal complaint. Even if the complaint cannot be resolved, the acknowledgment alone proves to the patient that the practice is interested in its patients' concerns.

Foster teamwork

Patients can readily perceive dysfunction in a medical practice, and it can play a large role in patient assessment of your telephone service. For example, if a telephone operator handles repeat calls from a patient throughout the day and informs the patient that it is the clinical staff's fault for not promptly returning his or her calls, telephone operators are sharing the internal dysfunction of a medical practice. The importance of teamwork should not be overlooked. The level of patient satisfaction typically mirrors the level of staff satisfaction. Make sure your medical practice is functioning as a true care team.

Message-taking Tools

Your employees need the skills and tools to take accurate and complete telephone messages. Telephone message pads should feature templates with boxes to check off (if manual) or point and click (if electronic) to improve message quality and staff efficiency. Everyone whose duties include answering a telephone should know basic medical terminology and be adept at correctly spelling important medical terms that describe chief complaints, diagnoses, medications, and other common medical issues. Indecipherable messages force you to call back patients, pharmacies, laboratories, or other physicians to figure out what they said. Returning calls to patients (or other callers) simply to request clarification of the initial message constitutes rework, which is costly for your medical practice. It also leads to caller frustration and the perception that your practice is inefficient. Rather than forwarding messages from one party to another, establish protocols to route messages—ideally automatically—to the person(s) who are accountable for handling them.

Why take a message?

The first important step to efficient message handling is to eliminate unnecessary messages whenever it is possible and appropriate to do so. For example, a scheduler can be delegated the authority to make a decision regarding a same-day visit request without having to take a message and run it by the physician. Nurses, medical assistants, and other clinical associates can be given their own business cards, which can be handed to patients along with a personal introduction and communication that he or she can provide needed assistance if the patient has questions, thereby avoiding unnecessary messages for providers. It's a small investment that helps create credibility. By empowering your staff, you reduce the time-consuming steps of taking, transmitting, and responding to messages, and, just as important, patients gain confidence in the practice.

Physicians can help this process along. A physician's verbal assurance to the patient that his or her clinical associate, or the practice's health coach or patient navigator, is an important member of your team helps patients feel comfortable communicating with a team member. This also reduces the volume of telephone calls by patients who state: "I only want to talk with my doctor." A team approach to patient care and to managing inbound calls is becoming the norm.

Finally, ask your staff members to sit down and record the questions that are most frequently asked of them. Gather the physician's input to the question, and organize the material in a notebook or electronic database that can be accessed by staff. (Note that generic nurse triage protocols are available for purchase in manual or electronic format; this purchase may replace your internal efforts—or supplement them.) With a database of protocols, staff can confidently respond to questions based on the written guidelines. Don't overstep the bounds of knowledge, however. If a patient has a question or need that is beyond the scope of expertise of the clinical assistant or nurse, they should not try to answer the question. But neither should they just revert to saying, "I need to ask Dr. Smith." Instead, respond: "That is an excellent question, Ms. Walters. I'd like to run that question by Dr. Smith. Where can I reach you when I call back?" Then query the physician, and call the patient back with a response in a timely manner.

Message completeness

Accurate and complete messages are essential to an efficient practice. In either paper or electronic templates, develop sample messages to respond to each of the following telephone inquiries:

- Test result requests;
- Medication renewals;
- Frequently asked questions of the nurse;

- Same-day appointment requests;
- Scheduling appointments when the patient has not been seen for a pre-defined period of time; and
- Other common requests to your practice.

During new employee training, review the sample messages, pointing out the essential components of each and make sure your staff members are consistently taking accurate and complete messages by auditing their messages in comparison to the samples. Train new employees on accessing your protocols and guidelines.

Use the telephone tracking worksheet discussed in Chapter 4 to focus on topics to educate staff members so they can improve their message-taking skills. Ensure that this education includes appropriate follow-up questions that employees should ask to determine the reason for the call and ensure that they garner sufficient detail about the issue. Develop scripts regarding common patient inquiries so that suitable follow-up questions and details are obtained for an accurate and complete message, and that an appropriate determination is made regarding the urgency of the call and its subject matter.

For the majority of calls, this step increases the likelihood that the call can be managed without the need for an outbound communication to the patient to request clarification.

Missed messages

Documentation of every telephone call is vital. Emphasize to staff and providers that every telephone call represents a patient's life. Failure to record a message is simply not acceptable. In addition to documenting all messages, ensure that all messages are responded to within a defined time period. With an EHR system, the message can be seamlessly integrated with the patient's record. In a paper system, however, tools are needed to make sure all messages are tracked. One method is to take messages on a duplex pad. Keep one copy with the pad, thereby creating a running log of all inbound calls. File the original message in the patient's chart by taping it inside the chart. Another method is to take messages on paper that has adhesive on one side to facilitate chart filing, while keeping a copy of the message in a folder in the event that the original is lost.

All communication must be documented and responded to; compliance is vital. Message-taking is a risk management issue that needs to be given high priority. Discuss your protocols with the practice administrator, medical director, and the director(s) assigned to internal risk management, as well as your malpractice carrier to make sure that your processes meet quality standards.

BEST PRACTICE

DOCUMENTATION AND APPROPRIATE MANAGEMENT OF EVERY TELEPHONE CALL ARE VITAL. EMPHASIZE TO STAFF AND PROVIDERS THAT EVERY TELEPHONE CALL REPRESENTS A PATIENT'S LIFE.

How to reach patients

A key step in taking a message is to determine how to return the caller's inquiry. When taking messages, urge staff to recognize the importance of accurately recording patients' telephone numbers to permit calls to be returned in a timely manner. Gather a "best" callback number from the caller, and always request an alternate as well. For example, "Is 555.555.5555 the best number to reach you at today? Is there another number that we can use to contact you in case we can't reach you at the first number you gave us?" Use the patient's call as an opportunity to review the telephone numbers on file for the patient. This allows your staff to perform a quick, but very helpful registration update to correct the telephone number in the registration portion of the patient's account. Integrate these same instructions via your patient portal, encouraging patients to document their message as well as the best method to return the communication.

> ### BEST PRACTICE
>
> Embrace communication methods that do not require synchronous work. The use of a patient portal, secure electronic message, or text message shifts work to platforms that are more efficient and minimizes inbound telephone calls.

As discussed in Chapter 5, proactively ask patients to use technology to communicate. During the message-taking and/or callback process, for example, providers and staff can encourage patients to use the practice's patient portal. Secure electronic and/or text messaging may also be an option, with the patient's written permission. These means of communication do not require synchronous communication; shifting work to platforms that are more efficient for your practice to manage minimizes telephone calls to and from your practice—and saves significant resources.

Alternatives to message-taking

If your employees are taking a high volume of messages, explore other avenues to manage calls without the need for a message. For example, use the management techniques we described in Chapter 5 to minimize inbound call demand. Or consider whether it is time for a telephone nurse triage and advice unit to directly manage clinical calls without the need for an initial step that involves a nonclinical person taking a message. Or perhaps your practice can create secure electronic messaging with patients to permit them to submit their inquiries in writing to the practice, thereby eliminating the need for a telephone call—and a message to be taken.

First-call resolution

To fundamentally improve efficiency and reduce resources that must be allocated to your telephones, set a goal of first-call resolution. Instead of taking a message and playing the game of telephone tag, develop a protocol so that callers' needs are met during their initial call. That is, the caller gets to the right person and his or her request for information is satisfied in real time. Indeed, the act of message taking is not an insignificant process. In fact, it is quite costly.

Our research reveals that each message, on average, costs $15, and other experts have estimated the cost to exceed $30 per message. At minimum, before a message is even taken, require staff members to ask: "Is there anything that I can do to help you?" Although not all calls can be resolved this way, this protocol definitely reduces the number of messages that must be taken. Staff training is an essential component of this strategy; the ability of the employee to provide accurate and thorough information, and to be competent at handling the patient's questions and problems, is a significant driver of patient satisfaction. First-call resolution is predicated on the ability of employees to be capable of handling the call to completion without requiring assistance via a transferred call or a subsequent call. Avoiding these transfers or subsequent calls translates into higher efficiency and better access service.

BEST PRACTICE

SET A GOAL OF FIRST-CALL RESOLUTION. EVERY MESSAGE COSTS YOUR PRACTICE, ON AVERAGE, $15.

Allowing the appropriate staff member to get the job done on the caller's first communication is perhaps the greatest asset that an EHR system can offer to your operations. With the patient's information immediately available, the needs of many callers—from patients to referring physicians—can be handled more expeditiously. If you have an EHR system, make sure you take advantage of the tools that maximize your practice's ability to provide first-call resolution to callers.

Callbacks

Callbacks is a term commonly used by practices to describe return calls to patients and other callers. To maintain the high-level customer service you expect to deliver, as well as to appropriately manage internal risk, the callback process needs to be effectively managed. Develop guidelines for providers and staff regarding call-backs, including:

- Protocols for physician-to-physician callbacks;
- Establishment and adherence to turnaround time for patient callbacks; and
- Protocols to enhance the use of technology.

These considerations are reviewed, in detail, in the sections that follow.

Physician-to-physician calls

To reduce callbacks to referring physicians, expedite physician-to-physician communication. The time it consumes to record a message from a physician who calls, route the message to the physician, allow the physician time to review the message, play telephone tag, and, finally, reach the originating physician not only adds delays to the process, but it also is very expensive—for both physicians! Several options can be considered as you work to streamline physician-to-physician calls.

Each staff member must make a judgment as to whether or not to interrupt the physician to take a telephone call. To avoid problems in varying judgments that may frustrate staff and providers, develop written guidelines as to if and when to interrupt the physician. Ensure that physicians agree with the guidelines and make sure the staff understands how to interpret the guidelines. Remember, every one of these calls is vital to your patients' care, so guidance is essential.

To streamline physician-to-physician communication, consider creating a separate telephone number or extension for referring physicians to use. Communicate this number to your referring physicians and determine one of the following methods to manage the inbound physician caller:

- The telephone (or extension) is immediately answered by the telephone operators, with the caller directly connected to the physician or that physician's nurse. The telephone system may be configured such that these calls are given priority in the queue.

- The telephone rings with a distinct tone at all stations in the suite (often referred to as a "bat telephone," red telephone, or presidential line) and each member of the staff is instructed to immediately answer those telephone calls if they are free to do so.

- A telephone with a distinct number or extension is held by a nurse (often rotating on a weekly basis); the nurse assigned to the telephone answers the call and discusses the immediacy of the issue with the physician caller.

- A telephone with a distinct number or extension is held by the physician on call who immediately responds to the caller.

- A telephone with a distinct number or extension is held by a physician; the responsibility is rotated among physicians on a weekly basis, thereby creating immediate access to a physician in the practice when referring physicians call.

- A central call center is established to process all inbound referring physician calls, particularly relevant for physician practices that are tasked with handling a very high volume of these calls.

We have witnessed successful implementation of each of the above options; however, as accountable care and collaborative care models are developed, the preferred model is to create a direct communication channel between physicians that does not rely on the synchronous communication required by the telephone. Instead, encourage referring physicians to correspond with your practice's physicians through a secure electronic method. This may be a part of the existing EHR system; a designated "e-Consult" platform; a community or health system–based health information exchange; a patient portal with functionality to accommodate referring physician communication; or perhaps a custom, secure electronic interchange engineered specifically for that purpose. Regardless of the platform, determining a better means of exchanging and documenting information between physicians should be a priority.

To reduce callbacks, as well as offer a value-added service, some medical

> ◆ **CASE STUDY** ◆
>
> **E-consults**
>
> DR. JOSEPH REECE, A PRIMARY CARE PHYSICIAN, SUSPECTS HIS PATIENT HAS BROKEN HER WRIST AND TAKES A DIGITAL X-RAY. HE COMMUNICATES WITH DR. SHUMAN, THE HAND SURGEON WHO IS ON CALL FOR VIRTUAL CONSULTS, TRANSMITTING THE CLINICAL DOCUMENTATION AND THE DIGITAL X-RAY TO THE SURGEON. TOGETHER, DRS. REECE AND SHUMAN DETERMINE THE NEXT STEPS FOR THE PATIENT.

practices have created an electronic consult capability. Let's review a case example of e-consults:

This e-consult—the availability of a physician assigned to provide consult capability on a given day—improves not only communication between physicians, but it also enhances the timeliness to care. It is likely that this model of physician-to-physician 'on-demand' communication will increase with time.

Callback protocols
Patients communicate with your medical practice every hour of every day. Message-taking, as discussed previously, is an important aspect of managing these calls, but those messages must not only be taken, but

also handled to fruition. To manage the calls, practices must establish and adhere to a turnaround time for patient callbacks.

Callbacks are not always handled in a timely manner. If the call isn't returned to the patient in a timeframe in which the patient believes is appropriate, the patient calls again. Repeat calls from patients are a significant source of opportunity for improvement, as patients initiate repeat calls to your practice when they do not receive a timely response to their initial inquiries. When the amount of staff time required to handle these calls is taken into account, repeat calls from patients can be a substantial, and mostly unnecessary, component of operating costs. Each of the following scenarios generates a high volume of repeat calls:

- Calls immediately go to voicemail; the caller is unsure if the message is picked up or when to expect a response.
- Patients are told to "give us a call to let us know how you are doing," but the message isn't retrieved. Thinking that the request is an important instruction, as it was communicated by their physician, patients call and call again trying to get through.
- A busy nurse doesn't check his or her voicemail until the end of the day. During the day, multiple messages from the same patient pile up.
- A message is taken by the telephone operator, but the caller does not have confidence that the operator understood his or her issue or took an appropriate message, so the patient calls back and leaves another message.
- A message is taken by the telephone operator; however, the caller has not been given a timeframe in which to expect a return telephone call.

> **BEST PRACTICE**
>
> ELIMINATE OR DRAMATICALLY REDUCE THE USE OF VOICEMAIL. VOICEMAIL IS SIMPLY A METHOD OF BATCHING AND DELAYING THE WORK. INSTEAD, CREATE REAL-TIME, ONE-TOUCH STRATEGIES TO RESPOND TO CALLERS.

Your medical practice can reduce the number of repeat calls from patients by implementing one or more of the following actions:

- Perform first-call resolution. Handle the patient's needs without having to take a message or call the patient back.
- Decrease the circumstances that lead to unnecessary calls.
- Eliminate or dramatically reduce the use of voicemail. Voicemail is simply a method to batch and delay work. Instead, create real-time, one-touch strategies that permit patients to receive information during their initial call.
- Separate the work of the patient visit from the work of the telephones, getting the telephones "off stage." As we discussed in Chapter 6: Telephone Staffing, this is the preferred model for staffing the telephones. This ensures that there is a dedicated, focused staff to manage the telephones, thereby reducing time delays and avoiding repeat calls.
- Ensure that telephone operators have the knowledge and communication skills to manage message-taking capability in a manner that engenders confidence. If not, the caller is likely to question the competency of the operator—the caller just does not have confidence that the operator took a complete message and gave it to the intended party, much less remembered to return the call when, or if, an answer is obtained. The result? The patient calls again, quite likely before the message has even reached the intended party.
- Inform the patient regarding when he or she should expect a return call. Meet with your staff and develop a standard

time frame by which all calls are returned. In this fashion, the caller is notified that he or she will receive a callback within three hours, for example, and can plan for that time delay. Then keep the service promise and be sure to place the return call to the patient within the three-hour window. Even if the inquiry is not resolved in that time frame, place the return call and notify the patient of the status of his or her inquiry. This helps prevent the person from calling back, again and again, asking the same question. Consider reviewing industry norms for callbacks when establishing your service expectations.

BEST PRACTICE

Establish a service promise—a turnaround time—for callbacks.

There's nothing more frustrating to a customer than unmet expectations. If you tell the patient to expect a test result in four days, then you need to communicate the result within those four days. Better yet, tell them to expect four days and then deliver in three days. Delight patients by setting appropriate expectations. Develop reasonable expectations that you can always beat by discussing the common timeframes that you will give to patients for test results notification, prescription renewals, surgery scheduling, referral processing, and physician or nurse callbacks. Distribute the expectations to providers and staff, and incorporate them into patient materials and your practice's website. Never set an expectation you can't beat. Exceeding your own expectations creates delighted customers; failing to meet them is a recipe for disaster.

Many medical practices have established a daily cutoff time for inbound communication. Patients who call or message the medical practice during the last hour of office hours are informed that unless the issue is urgent, they will not receive a return communication until the next business day. Note that many of these communications during the last hour are repeat calls or messages; the patient simply has not received a timely response and is now in limbo.

Although a cutoff time for callbacks is routinely used in many medical practices, it is likely not sustainable in the future as medical practices become part of accountable care networks, participate in patient-centered medical homes, and embrace similar value-based approaches to healthcare delivery. In place of the traditional 9-to-5 approach to patient access to nonemergency services, 24/7 access for patients is becoming the new, expected way of doing business. Feeding these expectations of instant access is the portability of healthcare information that an EHR system affords.

> **BEST PRACTICE**
>
> A CUTOFF TIME FOR CALLBACKS IS LIKELY NOT SUSTAINABLE IN THE FUTURE; 24/7 ACCESS CAPABILITY IS THE NEW, EXPECTED WAY OF DOING BUSINESS.

Some options to consider for your medical practice include:

- Work with your hospital to establish a 24/7 nurse triage line, with the nurse triage staff receiving access to the patients' medical records or working from established clinical protocols.
- Provide chronic care management services to align with the definition as reimbursed by insurers, or contract with a vendor dedicated to providing this service.
- Inform your answering service to transfer all calls at the end of day and after hours to a physician, advanced practice provider, or nurse from your practice who can respond to the patient in real time.
- Determine the need for an answering service; it may make more sense for your practice to have a nurse take "live calls" from patients at the end of the day or after hours. Studies have shown that when physicians give out their home or cellular telephone number to patients, it is rarely abused.

- Educate your patients so they can recognize the urgency of their medical situation. This enables them to understand the best action to take, for example, when a telephone call vs. a secure electronic message to the care team is most appropriate.
- Extend office hours to accommodate patients in the office, face to face. Seek remuneration for these visits, including the enhanced reimbursement that some insurance companies offer for after-hours care.[1]
- Establish performance expectations for all staff in the medical practice; if a call is received at the end of day, a staff member is given the responsibility to manage that call, including responding to the caller with an answer or a status update.
- Consider migrating your staff to an expanded workweek (for example, if they currently work 32 hours, expand to 36 hours) or flexing the hours of staff work (for example, variable shifts) to accommodate patients but avoid paying overtime.

In addition to calls from physicians and patients, your medical practice likely receives a high call volume from vendors, pharmacies, hospitals, and a host of other stakeholders. Managing callbacks to these entities depends on the urgency of the issue, as judged by the initial party who takes the call. Some of these calls will be transferred from a telephone operator to a nurse or manager to handle the issue, particularly if the call is of a clinical nature and urgent or time-sensitive. For example, the hospital admissions department has a question about a planned next-day admission or an important piece of equipment has broken and the vendor needs to determine whether a replacement unit is needed and when.

Other calls, however, are less urgent and a message can be taken and either sent to the appropriate inbox when electronic messaging is employed or a handwritten message can be taken and delivered to the party. For these calls, it is also important to establish a service expectation for the practice. For example, you may establish a policy that all non-physician or non-patient callers receive a callback no later than the end of the following day that their call is received. In this fashion, you can notify callers when to expect a return call, thereby avoiding repeat calls for the same issue—and at the same time position your practice for access and service delivery.

Take the opportunity to manage the callback process to avoid generating repeat calls. These calls tie up staff time unnecessarily and foster caller frustration—and even anger.

Summary

Your practice's access is evaluated each and every day by patients in the few minutes they interact with your staff via the telephone. Ensure that your employees have the tools they need to delight callers, to include telephone scripts and tools to enhance customer service, message-taking, and callbacks. Evaluate the work tools provided to the staff to identify opportunities to streamline work and/or leverage technology. Appropriate telephone call and message-handling tactics should become part of your practice's essential staff training and performance management process. Your efforts to eliminate repeat communication and optimize callbacks from your medical practice are critical to keeping your service promise.

End Note

1. See CPT codes 99050 and 99051. Comply with documentation and coding guidelines. CPT 2018 American Medical Association. All rights reserved.

CHAPTER 10

Systems and Technology

If telephone operations are on your mind, don't overlook the hardware and software of your telephone system. Managing the people and processes surrounding telephone access is important; however, achieving your goals is also dependent on the telephone system itself. Your telephone system may need new features or you may need to learn more about its existing features to optimize performance.

Several features for each telephone system need to be assessed. Although you may not need all of the functions that telephone system vendors offer, it's important to recognize the possibilities. As your practice changes, particularly if it is growing, it is likely that you will need to increase your system's functionality.

In this chapter, we discuss opportunities to understand and enhance the use of your telephone system to include:

- Effective voicemail and automatic call distributors (ACD) uses;
- Determining the considerations for selecting a system;
- Embracing opportunities to deploy telephony; and
- Recognizing the common functions available in a telephone system.

A multitude of functional options is now available for practices to employ in their telephone system; let's first review the most popular options: voicemail and the ACD.

Voicemail

Voicemail allows callers to communicate with employees at a time when they are busy or otherwise not available. The technology allows a caller to leave a verbal message in a voicemail box that can be later accessed by the user. The box is typically secured by a passcode that must be entered when the user wants to listen to the message.

Not everyone appreciates voicemail, however. Like an auto attendant, a complex voicemail system can easily frustrate callers. Even when you have the best intentions and the system is installed properly, voicemail can waste staff time, frustrate patients and referring physicians, and destroy your practice's service reputation.

If your medical practice decides to use voicemail, establish a written policy for it, including who, how, and when voicemail messages are retrieved. Exhibit 10.1 outlines a sample voicemail policy statement that you can use as a starting point for your medical practice. Establish a time frame for message retrieval, and monitor compliance with it. We recommend that all voicemail boxes be checked, at minimum, each hour. Each voicemail box should be assigned to a person who is accountable for managing the voicemail in accordance with the practice's expectations. All messages should be documented in the EHR system or in the practice's established messaging system. Define a specific process for recording information from voicemail into the patient's record or account and hold staff accountable to follow that process when handling voicemail responses.

BEST PRACTICE

IF YOU USE VOICEMAIL, CREATE FORMAL POLICIES AND PROCEDURES RELATED TO ITS USE. VOICEMAIL SHOULD BE USED SPARINGLY AND SHOULD NOT BE USED TO SCREEN CALLS OR AVOID ANSWERING THE TELEPHONES.

> **[EXHIBIT 10.1]** Voicemail sample policy statement
>
> **Policy Statement:** All telephones should be answered professionally, courteously, and promptly during normal business hours. Voicemail should be used sparingly, such as during high peak telephone demand and/or when a staff member is temporarily away from his or her work area. Voicemail should not be used to screen telephone calls or to avoid answering calls.

Greeting

Each voicemail greeting should be professional and brief, yet it should also provide enough information for the caller to make an informed decision regarding whether or not to leave a voicemail message. Include the following standard elements: professional greeting, name, information for urgent access, invitation for caller to leave a message, and expected response time. Account for the statements made in the automated attendant so as not to repeat the same information in the voicemail message.

> **BEST PRACTICE**
>
> BE SURE YOUR VOICEMAIL GREETING IS PLEASANT, APPROPRIATE IN TONE AND SPEED, AND CONCISE YET INSTRUCTIVE.

Sample voicemail greeting:

"Hello, this is Susan Green. I am Dr. Smith's nurse and you have reached my voicemail. If this is during normal working hours and you need immediate assistance, please dial "0" and ask for the operator. If you would like to leave a message, please leave your name, telephone number, and brief reason for your call, and I will return calls today between 1 and 5 p.m."

Alternatively, replace verbiage as appropriate: "If you would like to leave a message, kindly log on to our patient portal and send me a secure message."

Your greeting should be pleasant, appropriate in tone and speed, and concise yet instructive. For lines where patients may leave messages of a clinical nature, be sure the greeting message instructs patients to seek a live operator if the need is emergent or to dial 911 if the issue is potentially life threatening. (Check with your attorney or malpractice carrier for a recommended statement.) Of course, the prompts that patients hear should identify the person or department at which the caller is asked to leave his or her message. Update your voicemail greeting on a regular basis to ensure that the caller has the information needed to make an informed decision regarding whether or not to leave a voicemail based on your availability.

Retrieval and response

Staff members are responsible for retrieving voicemail promptly. Voicemail should be retrieved on a routine basis, preferably every 30 minutes and no less than once per hour. If the voicemail is from a patient or concerns a patient's care, the communication should be documented in the patient's record. The nature of the message should be recorded, as well as the time, date, and, if applicable, person who left the message. As with documenting any message, the caller's return telephone number should be recorded.

Responding to a voicemail, like any message, should be considered a priority. All telephone calls should be returned promptly within three hours unless the voicemail greeting indicates a longer absence. Even if the caller's issue has not been resolved, a return call should be made by the end of the three-hour period to inform the caller that the message has been received and to provide an update regarding the action that is planned or has been taken, with a new turnaround time provided to the caller. (See Chapter 9 for more information on callbacks.) If a nurse or medical assistant who maintains responsibility for calls is out for a period of time for leave or an unexpected absence, another staff member should be assigned the responsibility of managing these communications. It's ideal to establish "partners" or "teams" for staff members with duties related to communication. As patients' needs are not halted with the absence of a staff member, it's vital to cover all inbound communication channels every day.

Privacy

Callers have a right to a reasonable expectation of privacy. Voicemail messages should be considered confidential and should not be forwarded without the caller's permission.

Advantages and disadvantages

Is voicemail a time-saver or a time-waster in your practice? It's likely the latter if this 12-step scenario sounds familiar:

1. A patient calls your practice.

2. The receptionist who answers asks the caller to briefly describe her problem or question.

3. The receptionist transfers the patient to the correct staff member—in this case, a nurse.

4. Unfortunately, the nurse is elsewhere, so her voicemail answers the call.

5. The caller again describes her inquiry to the voicemail box.

6. After clinic concludes at 5:30 that evening, the nurse dials into the voicemail system to retrieve his messages.

7. He enters his password.

8. Then he wades through a menu of options, such as, "Press 1 for new messages" and "Press 2 to hear saved messages."

9. He listens to the patient's inquiry (often, a lengthy message during which he takes notes), noting that there are three messages from the same patient, each with a growing sense of urgency in the patient's voice. (If the receptionist who originally took the call also communicated a message, there would also be a fourth message for the nurse to review.)

10. He writes down the patient's telephone number—usually given at the very end of the message—and then deletes the messages from the system.
11. Then he calls the patient (add at least one more step if the nurse decides to assign the callback to someone else), but the patient is not at the callback number. He leaves a message.
12. Finally, the nurse gets the patient on the line and the entire inquiry is repeated. The patient is exasperated by having to leave multiple messages. By now, the patient has thought of a few more questions to ask, and, given the delay in response, is expecting a significant amount of time to be spent fulfilling her needs.

Voicemail, as in the previous scenario, is actually quite inefficient. Consider the time that you spend to access the system, to listen to the lengthy messages callers leave (and which they repeat again when you reach them), and, most importantly, the time it takes to track down the caller. One telephone call consumes countless minutes—minutes that you don't have to spare, and ones that only seem to frustrate callers.

Now, consider this alternative: the patient calls, asks a question, and you answer it. Sounds impossible? With an EHR system and a dedication to addressing the callers' needs right away, callers can be assisted on the initial response and first-call resolution can be performed because information is instantaneously accessible.

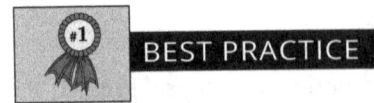

BEST PRACTICE

DEVELOP A GOAL OF FIRST-TIME RESOLUTION FOR ALL CALLS. THIS MAY REQUIRE CONSIDERATION OF HOW CALLS ARE ROUTED AND TO WHOM, BUT AVOIDING VOICEMAIL INCREASES EFFICIENCY AND PATIENT ACCESS TO YOUR PRACTICE.

Better yet, eliminate the demand for voicemail altogether by directing patients to message you via your secure electronic messaging system or through your patient portal. (See Chapter 5 for more tips on reducing the demand for telephone calls.) It's likely that voicemail will soon be a vestige of the past, like the rotary telephone, but it's an important process to manage wisely in the meantime.

If you are considering adding or expanding voicemail, first determine your needs and uses for it. Evaluate voicemail use for each functional area of your practice, including billing, referrals, scheduling, and clinical. Voicemail works best for the nonclinical functions of your practice, or at least those where there won't be an emergency that may lead to a bad outcome. These nonemergent uses for voicemail include billing, referral requests, and business issues. Although calls to these areas should be answered promptly, setting them aside for a short period should not lead to a risk management problem.

Regardless of the functional area, if you determine that voicemail is appropriate for an employee with telephone responsibilities, it should not be used to screen calls. Don't let staff use voicemail as a secretarial service. They may be on other calls, but in some cases they are just in the middle of another task or don't want the interruption of a call. Some might even purposely use voicemail to screen calls effectively blocking the patient's access to your practice. Make a simple rule: Pick up the telephone if you're not already on another call (and can't put that caller on hold to answer the other line or have it routed to an operator); use voicemail only when you're not available. Using voicemail for time-shifting—batching return calls to be made on your own time—doesn't increase efficiency. You actually end up busier than ever.

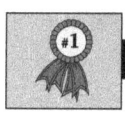

BEST PRACTICE

MAKE A SIMPLE RULE: PICK UP THE TELEPHONE IF YOU'RE NOT ALREADY ON ANOTHER CALL (AND CAN'T PUT THAT CALLER ON HOLD TO ANSWER THE OTHER LINE OR HAVE IT ROUTED TO AN OPERATOR); USE VOICEMAIL ONLY WHEN YOU'RE NOT AVAILABLE.

Some practices have banned voicemail. Employees are required to answer incoming calls and patients are rewarded with faster turnaround times for communicating via secure electronic messaging. An alternative to eliminating it altogether is to use it only during specific times, such as turning on the voicemail function during a staff meeting.

Basic functions

Determine how a voicemail system indicates that a message is waiting. Is there a blinking light, an LCD (liquid crystal diode) display, or other visual cue to tell you there's a new message in the system? Some systems can be integrated into the computer network to send alerts to assigned staff when new messages are waiting, with some systems even converting those voicemails to written messages using voice recognition software. Train staff and supervisors how to identify pending messages.

When choosing a voicemail system, consider its reporting capabilities. Sample activity reports should include the number of messages recorded, total length of messages, and average time before a message is deleted. These functions help you monitor the workload of your staff, as well as how your staff responds to messages from patients and referring physicians. Make sure that the system's port size and storage capacity are adequate for your needs. For example, how many messages can the voicemail system hold? How long of a message can callers leave?

What happens when the system is full? Will staff be alerted or must they depend on patients to tell them that a voicemail box is not accepting new messages? The more sophisticated the reporting, the more effective you will be at managing the system.

Choose a system with interactive voice response (IVR) software that recognizes and adapts to usage patterns. Sophisticated IVR systems can route calls from one of your top referring physicians, for example, directly to your clinical manager, or patients seeking directions straight to your location guidance. These advanced IVR systems can also identify callers based on the number that the caller is using, thus saving valuable time by reducing or eliminating the caller-identification process.

Avoid a stand-alone voicemail system because it does not allow users to return to a menu after they leave their voicemail message. As with a poorly designed auto attendant, voicemail that is not integrated with the rest of the telephone system may bounce users from an extension where no one picks up, then to the greeting message, back to another unattended extension, return to the greeting, and so on—a potentially endless cycle, and one that could drive away patients, referring physicians, and anyone else who calls. Always give callers an option to reach an operator instead of leaving a voicemail message.

Staff training

Training staff to use the system is as important as the system itself. When selecting a system, scrutinize the vendor's training materials in addition to checking references and the vendor's customer service reputation. Is online training, such as a web-based tutorial, available? Training materials should be comprehensive yet quick and simple to use. Include training on the voicemail system as a key component of new staff orientation. Make proficiency on the system a component of performance evaluations for the appropriate staff, as well as orientation for new staff.

Voicemail is a potential barrier to patient access and doesn't always increase practice efficiency-and may actually be harmful if improperly deployed. As you migrate communication away from the telephones to alternative communication channels, think of voicemail more as a back-up mechanism during peaks of heavy volume or special circumstances. Make voicemail work for you, not against you.

Automatic Call Distributor

An automatic call distributor (ACD)—or a product with similar functionality called a uniform call distributor (UCD)—distributes incoming calls within the practice. The ACD software recognizes busy lines and places callers in waiting queues, distributing the calls to specific lines when they become free. Essentially, an ACD creates the opportunity for you to better route, handle, and categorize calls without requiring an operator to do so. A closely related technology, the automated attendant, allows the telephone call to be "answered" automatically before it is routed through the distribution system.

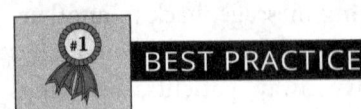

> **BEST PRACTICE**
>
> SPEND TIME PLANNING FOR YOUR AUTOMATIC CALL DISTRIBUTOR. IT CAN CREATE THE OPPORTUNITY TO BETTER ROUTE, HANDLE, AND CATEGORIZE CALLS; HOWEVER, IT CAN ALSO BACKFIRE AND FRUSTRATE CALLERS IF IT IS NOT WELL MANAGED.

An ACD, combined with an automated attendant, replaces the need for a staff member to respond and route telephone calls. After listening to a greeting and instructions, callers can route calls themselves by choosing options such as "Press 1 to schedule an appointment," "Press 2 to renew a prescription," "Press 3 to request a test result," and so forth. Callers and internal users should be able to identify and reach their destinations easily in just one or two steps.

When unmanaged, ACDs can backfire, just like poorly executed voicemail systems. One way in which these systems may backfire results when an internal stakeholder overreacts to the negative responses of what is often a small, but vocal, subset of patients who are unhappy with the automation in general. A physician or employee may react by giving out the practice's "backline" telephone number. Before long, the "back line" becomes a main line. Thus, the technology's cost savings are never realized as the practice struggles to manage these new, unexpected points of telephone entry.

Although many patients expect to encounter ACDs and attendants when calling credit card companies, banks, airlines, and government offices, they place higher demands on their physician's practice. Patients interact with their physicians on a much more personal level than they do with other businesses, and they are disappointed when it sounds like a computer is answering their physician's telephone. As time goes by, more patients are adjusting to this reality of a modern medical practice—unless, that is, the technology is executed poorly. Even so, practices in rural areas where small, independent medical practices are still the norm or those with a large senior patient panel might continue to reject this technology because too many of their patients feel it is impersonal and difficult to use. Of course, if you have the resources to invest, using a staff member to personally greet and respond to callers, as well as to distribute their calls, is ideal.

When evaluating ACD systems, be sure to understand the storage capabilities of the system and what happens to call overflow as well as the features listed in Exhibit 10.2.

ACD options

If you decide to use an ACD and attendant, create a clear and concise greeting and limit the number of options to avoid confusing the caller. We recommend the following:

> *Thank you for calling Medical Practice Associates. If this is an emergency, please hang up and dial 911. Please press one of the following options so we can best direct your call to meet your needs:*
>
> *Press 1:   To schedule or cancel an appointment*
> *Press 2:   To renew a prescription*
> *Press 3:   To request a test result*
> *Press 4:   To speak with a nurse*
> *Press 5:   To discuss your bill*
>
> *Please press 0 for all other calls or to speak with an operator.*

Practices may be able to combine options 2, 3, and/or 4. If more options are needed, consider sub-menus so that the main choices are limited to five. However, limit the sub-menu to one per choice so that callers can reach their destination with no more than two menu options.

We recommend that you list no more than five options so callers don't lose track—and patience. Moreover, if using sub-menus, recognize that the patient should not have to choose more than two options to reach a live person. Patients do not get mad at automated attendants; they get mad at feeling trapped and not reaching the right person.

Using the selections, a caller should be able to route his or her call to a staff member or staffing unit responsible to manage calls in each specific area with the goal of first-call resolution. Calls that are included on the options menu should be either directed to a specific person(s) or a different strategy should apply; don't fall into the trap of using this technology to simply count your call types.

BEST PRACTICE

LIST NO MORE THAN FIVE OPTIONS ON YOUR AUTOMATED ATTENDANT; AND IF USING SUB-MENUS, THE CALLER SHOULD NOT HAVE TO CHOOSE MORE THAN TWO OPTIONS TO REACH A LIVE PERSON.

[EXHIBIT 10.2] Features of an ACD

- Expandability
- Flexibility
- Wallboard support (displays incoming calls on a screen)
- Operators can transfer callers to an auto attendant
- Callers can opt in or out of 'queue' (and return to a live operator or another menu)
- Silent monitoring
- Operators can log in and out
- Report generation

Furthermore, provide frequent callers a number that moves them to the right party from the beginning of the call. For example, give referring physicians a specific number that moves them directly to a live person. Consider promoting a campaign such as "Dial 9 to save time" for referring physicians to ensure that the adoption of an ACD doesn't prevent their calls from being handled expeditiously.

BEST PRACTICE

> PATIENTS DON'T GET MAD AT AUTOMATED ATTENDANTS; THEY GET MAD AT FEELING TRAPPED AND NOT REACHING THE RIGHT PERSON. BEFORE GOING LIVE ON THE SYSTEM, TEST THE TECHNOLOGY AND MAKE SURE IT IS WORKING AS INTENDED.

For your prompts, don't use an automated voice, ask a staff member (or hire a professional) who has a positive voice presence to record the greeting and options. Importantly, be sure that your options are presented in order. Consider offering choices to non-English-speaking callers, depending on your patient population. Before you go live, test the technology yourself.

If you have determined that the technology isn't right for your general telephone line, consider its application for other situations such as in the business office, as a "back-up" for busy operators, for personal calls to staff members, or for reaching a referral coordinator.

Voicemail can be integrated with an ACD and attendant, allowing callers to leave a message at their chosen option if the requested staff member is unavailable. If you choose this option, make sure it's user-friendly and allows your callers to choose "0" to reach the operator because some people prefer to speak to an operator or don't know which option they should choose.

System Selection

When selecting a new telephone system, involve all stakeholders who use the technology. Develop a formal evaluation process to assess each of the vendors that you investigate.

Selecting or changing your system

A telephone system is a critical component of your management information systems. Don't limit your assessment; your telephone system deserves the same level of scrutiny that you exercise when selecting a practice management or EHR system.

Complete these steps before selecting or changing your telephone system:

- Learn telephone system terms and procedures. Like the healthcare industry, the telecommunications market is full of acronyms and technical terminology. Familiarizing yourself with the nomenclature keeps you on equal footing with your potential vendors. Exhibit 10.3 lists common terms associated with telephone systems and a brief definition of each.
- Learn the basic telephone equipment structure. Knowing the system's parts and features improves the outcome of your system evaluation process.
- Define your practice's needs. Review your existing system, as well as the features of the potential new system. Do you want better reporting, an enhanced ability to route or transfer callers, or extra features like automatic call distribution? Identify the specific features needed for your practice.
- Involve your staff. Speaking with all of your staff members to discuss specific needs, functions, and ideas for functionality, helps you choose the right system for your practice.
- Network with other practices of similar size and structure. Reach out to at least three colleagues to inquire about their systems—and the advantages and disadvantages of each.

- Gather information and proposals from vendors. Select three to five vendors to submit a request for proposal for your telephone system. The more specific you are, the more information you will garner from the proposals.

- Do your homework. Before you establish a relationship with the company that will manage your communications, investigate the vendors. Deal only with quality vendors, and require proof that they have the bandwidth to handle the volume of communications from your practice. The telephone is your main communication channel to external customers

> [EXHIBIT 10.3] Common features of telephone systems
>
> **Automated (auto) attendant:** A system that answers and routes calls after prompting callers. For example, "Thank you for calling Medical Practice Associates. If this is an emergency, please hang up and dial 911. Please press one of the following options so that we can best direct your call to meet your needs: press 1 to schedule or cancel an appointment; press 2 to renew a prescription; press 3 to request a test result; press 4 to speak with a nurse; press 5 to discuss your bill. Please press 0 for all other calls or to speak with an operator."
>
> **Automatic call distributor (ACD) or uniform call distributor (UCD):** Software products that help telephone operators better manage incoming calls by distributing calls evenly to staff, pointing callers to specific functions (for example, appointment requests and prescription renewals), and placing callers on automatic hold—"in queue"—until a staff member is available to take the call. ACDs or UCDs can be used in place of or as a back-up for your receptionist.
>
> **Call accounting:** Software programs that capture, record, analyze, and organize call data. The information is stored in a database that can be queried for operator productivity, call abandonment rate, and other analyses.
>
> **Call forwarding:** A function that allows you to program the system to ring elsewhere if a station is busy or a call is not answered within a predetermined number of rings. Some systems permit external forwarding; some forward only within the system.
>
> **Call hunt:** A function that bounces incoming calls automatically to the next available (not busy) line.
>
> (continues)

> **EXHIBIT 10.3** Common features of telephone systems (continued)

Call park: A function that allows you to place callers "in orbit," removing them from general telephone traffic to alert staff that a call is waiting.

Call transfer: A function that allows calls received from internal or external callers to be sent from one telephone to any other within the system.

Caller identification (ID): A function that allows you to identify the caller's registered name and number.

Capacity: The number of telephones, lines, and software that a telephone system can handle. For example, a 24-port system can handle a combination of 24 lines and telephones.

Central processing unit (CPU): The main cabinet that houses the telephone system's intelligence and controls its activities.

Custom call routing (CCR): A function that enables you to design custom routing points for callers—a big plus offered by some auto attendants. For example, a caller can leave a message in a mailbox and then be routed to specific locations within a business.

Direct inward dialing (DID): A function that enables a caller to bypass the receptionist and be routed directly to the desired extension. DID trunks are assigned through the telephone company. Each trunk ordered has 24 associated telephones, each of which can be assigned to individual staff members.

Interactive voice response (IVR): Software that prompts callers for information by asking them to use their telephone keypads or, in some systems, utter certain phrases in response to automated questions. IVR improves staff efficiency by routing callers to the appropriate staff based on information the caller provides.

Intercom: A function that enables you to ring another telephone within the system and talk internally without tying up an outside line.

Port: A port is the point of connections in a system. Consider this the interface point at which programs are routed into the telephone system. A two-port voicemail system enables two activities; a four-port voicemail system allows four; an eight-port, eight. Ports are avenues that are open for travel when connected to a CPU.

(continues)

> [EXHIBIT 10.3]   Common features of telephone systems (continued)

Predictive dialer: A system focused on managing outbound calls, this technology automatically dials batches of telephone numbers for connection to staff. Based on parameters established by management, these systems adjust the calling process to the number of staff members it anticipates (or predicts) will be available when the calls being placed are expected to be answered. The predictive dialer discards unanswered calls, engaged numbers, disconnected lines, answers from fax machines, voicemail and similar automated services, and only connects staff to the calls that are actually answered by people. This technology practically eliminates wasted staff time by connecting telephone operators with a live person immediately.

Remote notification: A pager or cellular phone notifies the user that he or she has a voicemail message.

T1: A digital transmission link with a capacity of 1.544 Mbps (1,544,000 bits of data per second). T1 normally can handle 24 simultaneous voice conversations or data links over two pairs of wires, each one digitized at 64 Kbps. This is accomplished by using special encoding and decoding equipment at each end of the transmission path to multiplex one circuit into 24 channels. The next generation of this technology, T2 and T3 lines, carries multiple T1 channels multiplexed, resulting in higher transmission rates (6.312 and 44.736 Mbps, respectively).

Telephony: The use or operation of an apparatus or device for the transmission of sounds between distinct, separate points (can be with or without connecting wires).

Traffic: The number of users on a call.

Trunk: A line or telephone number.

Voice over Internet protocol (VoIP): A technology that enables routing of voice conversations over the Internet or any other IP network. The voice data flows over a general-purpose packet-switched network instead of the traditional dedicated, circuit-switched voice transmission lines. Also referred to as IP telephony and Internet telephony.

Wireless telephone: A portable telephone that can fully integrate into your system and can be used from anywhere in your office.

(patients and referring physicians), as well as your internal network.

- Understand your patients. No matter what features or applications you consider, keep in mind the needs of your patient population. Pay special attention to the design of an automated system if large numbers of your patients are not used to dealing with automated telephones or if English is not their primary language.

Analyze the investment

After the telephone system (or a new feature, enhancement, or software product) is installed, gauge where it works and does not work. Spend a few minutes each day in your reception area asking patients for their opinions. Obtain feedback from your key referring physicians and their staff. Be sure to solicit advice from the staff at your entire practice, as it affects everyone from the receptionist to the physicians, as well as your patients. Ask: Is it effective? Has it saved you time and/or money? Has it made your practice more efficient? Has it decreased or increased your response time to patients? Is your "return on investment" positive? If not, what steps can you take to improve the system?

Expect to use the system for at least six weeks before you see any impact on response times and costs. If the answers to the above questions are a resounding "no" for a particular feature, such as an ACD, then don't invest in an ACD and attendant, particularly if you can place your efforts into directing patients to communicate with you via secure electronic messaging or a patient portal instead.

Consider workflow

Map your practice's workflow to ensure that this new technology is used efficiently. Your callers, regardless of where or how the call is routed, should receive a timely response.

Choose with care

Carefully select the product and the vendor. Study the vendor's track record. Talk to several other practices that use the system. Negotiate a trial period to test the system, and don't skimp on service or training. Are all of these cautions really necessary? Yes! Your patients may never forgive you for losing their calls, and you may place your practice into a risk management situation.

BEST PRACTICE

INVESTIGATE TELEPHONY APPLICATIONS THAT INTEGRATE WITH YOUR SYSTEMS TO PLACE OUTBOUND CALLS TO PATIENTS—SUCH AS APPOINTMENT REMINDERS—FREEING UP TELEPHONE STAFF FOR TASKS THAT ARE KNOWLEDGE INTENSIVE.

Telephony applications

Telecommunications software products (referred to collectively as telephony applications) are now readily available for use in a medical practice. These software products integrate with your information systems to replicate or back up services that your practice currently provides. For example, you can purchase appointment confirmation systems that integrate with your practice management system (the scheduling module, in particular). These systems access the schedule for the following day and initiate calls and/or text messages to remind patients of their appointments. The software finds the telephone numbers associated with each patient's name and places outbound calls or texts to those numbers to communicate a reminder for the patient's upcoming appointment. Systems can be established to call only the patient's primary telephone number or they can work through the alternate telephone numbers the patient has provided for appointment reminders. In addition to appointment confirmations, telephony applications can assist practices with a multitude of functions, many of which are highlighted in Exhibit 10.4.

Other considerations

In addition to the configuration of a system's key functions, there are a host of other factors to consider when selecting or implementing a telephone system. Evaluate the following issues as you refine your telephone system.

Discuss compliance with current federal and state regulations regarding telephony applications with your lawyer, to include the FCC's 2015 ruling regarding automated appointment reminders.

> We grant the exemption...but restrict it to calls for which there is exigency and that have a healthcare treatment purpose, specifically: appointment and exam confirmations and reminders, wellness checkups, hospital pre-registration instructions, preoperative instructions, lab results, post-discharge follow-up intended to prevent readmission, prescription notifications, and home healthcare instructions...(FCC, *Telephone Consumer Protection Act Omnibus Declaratory Ruling and Order*, released July 10, 2015.)

Consideration of current regulations is important regarding the content of telephony-based communication with patients, as well as the delivery.

If your practice provides services that may be considered sensitive (such as psychiatry, obstetrics, oncology, and infectious disease), consider blocking your practice's "caller identification (ID)" when calling patients. Without blocking, your practice's name and number may appear on the recipient's caller ID display when you call patients to remind them of appointments or report that test results have arrived. This identification could compromise the patient's confidentiality if others in the household or business see it. Instead, consider using a number that remains unidentified, often displaying as "private caller" or "unknown" on recipients' telephones. Many practices have begun to use this feature to avoid patients automatically dialing the number back (an almost instantaneous process on most cellular phones, which create a trail of 'missed calls' that can be redialed with a swipe of the finger), before listening to your message or even when no message is left. Avoid a specific identification of one particular area of your practice—the business office—on your caller ID. If the name 'business office' appears on your patients' cellular phones when one of your staff members calls, there's no guarantee that any patient will respond to your call.

[EXHIBIT 10.4]   Telephony applications

- Appointment reminders and confirmations
- Test results reporting
- Collection calls
- Patient educational material requests
- Pre-recorded patient instructions and explanations
- Prescription requests
- Staff notifications
- Patient satisfaction surveys

While patients are waiting on hold or being transferred, use the opportunity to deliver custom messages about your practice. After being placed on hold, the patient is essentially captive. Avoid blank space or elevator music; instead, use on-hold messaging to communicate important information that provides value to your patients—and your practice. For example, record a message with an invitation to register for your patient portal. Or use the opportunity to disseminate information regarding vaccine availability and flu shots. Alternatively, you may announce the addition of a new provider. You can also focus on disseminating information about services you offer or supplement your message with answers to frequently asked questions. The best sources to discover these common questions are your staff and telephone logs (see Chapter 4). Key in on the subjects that produce the highest call volume where staff members are essentially repeating the same message over and over to callers. In addition to saving staff time, you may be able to reduce the number of future incoming calls requesting this information.

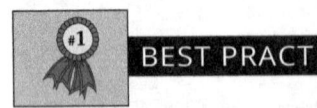

> **BEST PRACTICE**
>
> WHILE PATIENTS ARE WAITING ON HOLD, USE THE OPPORTUNITY TO DELIVER CUSTOM MESSAGES ABOUT YOUR PRACTICE, SUCH AS AN INVITATION TO REGISTER FOR YOUR PATIENT PORTAL AND INFORMATION ABOUT NEW PROVIDERS OR SERVICES.

Summary

If you need to select a new telephone system or change the capabilities of your current system, use the same intense scrutiny as you would when selecting a practice management or EHR system. Deploy your best efforts to match a system's capability with your practice's telephone access demand. Buying new equipment, by itself, isn't the sole answer to keeping telephone demand in check. Before shopping for new technology, examine your current processes to see where you can change telephone management or even reduce telephone demand. Then, by enhancing your operations and deploying technology, you can begin to help yourself—and your patients—to focus more of your days on improving health and less of it on answering telephones.

CHAPTER 11

Key Performance Indicators

As part of your patient access strategy, it is business critical to develop and monitor key performance indicators related to patient access. Business intelligence about patient access should populate a dashboard that reports your practice's goals for each aspect of access and the performance related to each of these variables. Sharing these measures practice-wide helps educate providers and employees on patient access issues, as well as areas of success and opportunity.

Consider integrating patient access measures in your dashboard to permit ongoing tracking and monitoring of performance. Revisit the measures at routine intervals and ensure that the measure and its operational definition, as well as the target for your medical practice, are appropriate.

BEST PRACTICE

AS PART OF YOUR PATIENT ACCESS STRATEGY, DEVELOP PATIENT ACCESS GOALS FOR YOUR MEDICAL PRACTICE THEN CREATE A DASHBOARD THAT REPORTS YOUR PRACTICE'S PERFORMANCE FOR EACH OF THESE GOALS.

Exhibit 11.1 reports the measure, its operational definition, how to calculate the measure and a recommended target. Although we have cited targets, the most important consideration is what your patients want and need. Gather feedback from your patients and referral physicians, gain knowledge about your market and discuss your own expectations for patient access based on clinical guidelines adopted by your providers.

[EXHIBIT 11.1] Key performance indicators

Measure	Operational Definition	Calculation	Target
Capacity/fill rate	The loss of provider capacity as measured by the number of visit slots available and the number of arrived visits.	The number of arrived patient visit slots divided by the number of available patient visit slots.	Greater than 95%.
New patient lag time	The number of days that new patients wait for their appointment.	The calendar days between the date of the patient's request and the actual date of the appointment.	14 day average. Less or more time defined by service/diagnosis.
Established patient lag time	The number of days that established patients wait for their appointment.	The calendar days between the date of the patient's request and the actual date of the appointment.	Acute needs: same day to primary care; two days to specialty care. Non-acute needs: 10 to 14 days (may be variable by specialty).
New patient growth	New patients as a percentage of total patients.	The number of new patients arrived divided by the total number of arrived patients.	20–40% for growing (versus mature) practices. May be variable by specialty.
Patients scheduled but not arrived	Percentage of patients scheduled but not arrived.	The number of patients who failed to keep their appointment (to include cancellations, bumped, now shows) divided by the number of patients scheduled.	Less than 20%.

(continues)

[EXHIBIT 11.1] Key performance indicators (continued)

Measure	Operational Definition	Calculation	Target
Appointment no-show rate	The percentage of appointments that patients fail to keep.	The number of patients who were a no-show for their appointment divided by the total number of appointments. Do not include cancellations or bumps.	Less than 8%.
Appointment "bump" rate	The percentage of appointments that the provider cancels in which patients must be bumped.	The number of patient visits that the provider cancels divided by the number of visits scheduled.	Less than 2%.

It is important to recognize that although these patient access metrics are invaluable to a medical practice to determine its ability to balance provider supply and patient demand, it is difficult to obtain an accurate measure of patient demand. Your daily visit schedule only defines the patients who were successful in reaching your practice, being serviced by one of your schedulers, and making it through your scheduling process. Consider that your real demand may be vastly different from your scheduling system. Indeed, some prospective patients may have a difficult time navigating your scheduling process. In frustration based on the scheduling process—or when faced with appointment availability that is not consistent with their expectations, patients may pursue other options, to include abandoning their call when placed on hold, and/or indicating they will call back (but never do).

Thus, the patient demand that is identified in your measures may only be a subset of true demand for your services. Unless and until measures related to ease of access (via the telephone or self-scheduling) are also evaluated, 'leakage' of patients to the community may be occurring without your knowledge.

In addition to the metrics outlined in Exhibit 11.1, it is important to measure and monitor your telephone performance. Exhibit 11.2 reports key performance metrics to track and monitor related to telephone access. These measures were discussed in Chapter 4 of this book. Evaluate your practice's performance in each of these areas to determine telephone access opportunity.

Beyond telephone access, establish measures that are relevant to the other access channels that your practice has deployed. These may include one or more of the following:

- Volume of patient portal registrations;
- Percentage of active patients who have registered for the patient portal;
- Utilization of active patients related to each function (for example, prescription renewal requests) offered by the patient portal;
- Percentage of messages that are self-served;
- Average (or median) number of hours to respond to messages;
- Percentage of new patient appointments that are self-scheduled;
- Percentage of established patient appointment that are self-scheduled;
- Volume of referrals received via the online request, health information exchange, or other technology platform;
- Average (or median) number of hours to convert appointment requests to scheduled appointments; and
- Percentage of the business day in which the web chat function is available.

As the channels to access your practice diversify, incorporate performance metrics for each one to monitor the success of your investment.

EXHIBIT 11.2 Performance expectations for quality metrics

Measurement	Expectation
Abandonment rate	3% or less
Availability	85% or more, based on workday unless excused for training or other duties
Average handle time	Set in accordance with practice protocols; monitored by management with a focus on after-call employee efficiency
Average speed to answer	24 seconds or less (maximum of four rings, if manually calculated)
Callback rate	Clinical: Within 30 minutes of initial call. All others: All calls acknowledged within three hours of receipt, regardless of ability to fully answer the request. Answer by end of day, unless extenuating circumstances. 100% of callbacks made, and performed within established time frames.
Duration of call	Set in accordance with practice protocols; monitored by management but not a component of employee performance
Hours of operation	30 minutes before office hours begin until 5 p.m. Open continuously through the lunch period.
Message quality	100%
On-hold time	30 seconds or less
Script compliance rate	100%
Service	100% professionalism, courtesy, compassion, and empathy; use of service recovery
Service level	80% within 30 seconds
Staff occupancy	80% or more, but depends on size of operation and expected performance quality
Trunk blockage	0%

Create market awareness

Determine the appointment lag times of the competitors in your market to ensure that access to your practice meets or exceeds the expectations regarding availability of patients and referring physicians. Notably, the concept of 'market' depends on your specialty. A primary care provider may pull from a 10-mile radius, whereas a pediatric neurologist may pull from a state or multi-state area.

Assess new patient accommodation opportunities

Today, patients can readily 'shop' for appointments online. These offerings allow patients to be accommodated through a platform made available by a practice (or a health system on behalf of each of its practices) or a third-party vendor that contracts with a practice to provide the functionality. Typically, the platform is integrated with the practice's practice management system, with the offering acting as a clearinghouse to view the appointment calendars of physicians (based on slots that are 'released' for this purpose), and the insurance plans that are accepted. For the vendor which provides the platform, practices may pay a flat monthly fee or an assessment per scheduled appointment. Instead of rejecting this new marketplace, practices have recognized the value of this new channel to attract patients, as well as the opportunity to fill empty appointment slots.

This instantaneous electronic access to the provider's schedule is a far cry from the telephone holds and telephone tags often involved in patient scheduling.

Master Quality Payment Program access metrics

Many of the improvement activities outlined by the Centers for Medicare and Medicaid Services' Quality Payment Program (QPP) for medical practices feature patient access. Consider evaluating these access measures as a starting point for your patient access initiative. By adopting these measures, a medical practice can focus on patient access while at the same time 'earning' the points needed for differential reimbursement in the QPP. Some of the improvement activities involving patient access include:

- Collection of patient experience data on access to care and development of an improvement plan.
- Providing specialist reports back to the referring clinician to close the referral loop.
- Timely communication of test results.
- Regular care coordination training.
- Tracking specialist-referred patients through the entire process.
- Access to enhanced patient portal to provide updated clinical information with interactive and bidirectional features.

Summary

Identify your patient access goals and measure and monitor your performance on a systematic basis. This will help build a culture of access and provide early warning signs to alert you to access opportunities in your practice.

Conclusion

Patient access is the lifeline of any medical practice. Use this book as a blueprint to develop the strategic goals and tactical plans to improve access to your practice and meet patient demand.

Focus on your capacity to meet patient demand and work to expand capacity if this is needed. Develop specific patient access targets and measure your performance as you work to cultivate a culture of access in your practice.

Make sure patients can easily make an appointment with your providers. The scheduling methods and optimization tools provided in this book will help to expand patient access and streamline your patient flow process. Importantly, scheduling optimization is a prerequisite for expanding capacity while optimizing the provider's time.

Since patients and referring physicians continue to rely on the telephone to seek appointments, redesign, and staff your telephones for optimal performance. Embrace the tools in this book, including telephone scripts, message-taking, callbacks, and communication tools to help your staff members become experts in telephone management.

Given the importance of patient access, evaluate the need for a focused call center to manage both the business and clinical calls to your practice. This virtual front office will ensure a consistent level of service, knowledge and expertise provided to patients. If you decide to embark on a call center, use the development and management tools for access centers described in this book as a guide to staff your own virtual front office.

We also encourage you to develop the infrastructure, tools and technology platform needed for virtual communication, virtual access and telehealth services. "If you build, it they will come" is transformed into "care anywhere, anytime." These newer access strategies are expected to become integrated with traditional episodic visits as we further the journey to value-based care.

Index

A
Abandonment rate, 45-48, 64, 109, 114, 115, 119, 125, 152, 157, 215, 227
Access center, 124, 129, 131, 230
Access metrics, 4, 7, 52, 224, 228
Action plan, 34, 62-64, 83, 101
Advanced access scheduling, 16, 65, 66, 165
Agent routing, 142, 143, 145
Appointment reminder, 70, 220
Automatic Call Distributor (ACD), 40, 142, 201, 210, 215
Average handle time, 46, 47, 109, 154, 227

B
Basic forecast, 135
Billing, 33, 42, 90-91, 97, 113, 124, 152, 207
Bump, 10-11, 30-31, 66, 68, 224-225
Business calls, 113-114

C
Call center, 2, 45, 47, 50, 123-158, 192, 195, 230
Call demand, 33-59, 61-63, 73, 80, 87-88, 108, 113-114, 131, 134, 164, 189
Call leveling, 145-147
Call type, 63, 135-136, 153-154, 170, 212
Call volume, 35-46, 48-49, 59, 61-64, 76, 81, 86, 96, 101, 103, 105, 108, 112, 115-117, 133-139, 144-146, 198, 221
Callback, 48, 55, 105, 146, 153, 181, 188, 190, 192-193, 195-199, 205-206, 230
Callback rate, 46, 48, 227
Call-handling, 51-52
Cancellation, 10, 16, 19, 25-26, 29-31
Case studies, 5-6, 112, 114, 193
Clinical calls, 48, 80-82, 84-85, 108, 113-114, 117-118, 146, 189, 230
Clinical mentoring, 13
Closing, 54, 170, 174
Communication tools, 169, 178, 230
Complaints, 10, 149, 182-184
Culture of access, 4, 229-230

D
Downtime, 112, 133, 136-137
Duration of call, 46, 49, 227

E
Erlang C method, 135, 136, 137

F
Focused planning, 152

G
Gap analysis, 59
Greeting, 105, 170, 173-174, 203, 209-211, 213

H
Hiring, 24, 57, 61, 101, 104, 106-107, 113
Hiring philosophy, 106

I
Inbound call tracking, 42
Inbound call volume 36, 37, 38, 40, 49, 59, 86, 96, 101, 108, 115
Integration, 151, 152, 153, 155

233

L

Lag time, 7, 8, 12, 13, 25, 29, 30, 67, 224, 228
Level load, 23, 24

M

Modified wave scheduling, 16

N

No-show, 10, 16, 19, 28, 29, 30, 31, 69, 225

O

On deck, 93
On-hold time, 46, 49, 50, 221, 227
Outbound calls, 41, 43, 61, 62, 63, 68, 70, 79, 86, 94-95, 123, 126, 133, 136, 138, 153, 217, 219, 220

P

Patient access opportunity, 2, 28
Patient advisory, 52, 57
Patient portal, 31, 44, 64, 68, 70, 71, 72, 75, 84, 86, 90, 92, 95, 96, 97, 123, 147, 161, 163, 164, 172, 188, 192, 204, 207, 219, 221, 226
Performance indicators, 2, 7, 36, 52, 223-229
Performance management, 103, 119, 171, 199
Performance measures, 35
Permission (results), 17, 72, 73, 110, 188, 205
Pharmacy, 6, 63, 74, 75, 79, 131
Planned care visit, 82, 83, 86
Prescription, 30, 33, 74, 75, 76, 77, 78, 79, 113, 116, 123, 126, 129, 131, 152, 171, 196, 210, 211, 215, 220
Prime appointment, 28
Productivity threshold, 145
Provider shortages, 3, 162

R

Reimbursement reform, 163
Response sets, 175

S

Scheduling horizon, 30, 67, 68
Scheduling template, 5, 13, 16, 17, 66, 67, 68
Scripts (scripting), 46, 51, 52, 57, 64, 93, 116, 120, 125, 147, 148, 169-171, 175, 183, 186, 199
Self-scheduling, 68, 69, 97, 225
Service level, 45, 48, 50, 109, 114, 125, 132, 137, 140, 152, 153, 227
Service promise, 181, 195, 196, 199
Shop for care, 29, 228
Single interval scheduling, 15, 16
Social media, 84, 92, 108, 126, 161
Speed to answer, 45, 46, 47, 48, 57, 109, 114, 125, 127, 152, 227
Staff occupancy, 46, 50, 51, 227
Staff workload, 109, 110, 114
Stage/staging, 19, 77, 78, 115, 118, 154, 194
Stakeholders, 3, 4, 7, 13, 79, 124, 128, 156, 157, 158, 161, 198, 210, 214

T

Telephony applications (TAPI), 68, 105, 219-220
Telephone management, 1, 2, 35, 38, 43, 45, 52, 63, 66, 94, 104, 112, 120, 128, 132, 138, 222, 230
Telephone staff, 47, 49, 58, 64, 71, 75, 103-122, 124, 177, 180, 194
Telephone staffing model, 108
Telework, 140, 141
Tipping point (appointment time), 30
Transfers, 63, 65, 96, 100, 189, 205
Transitions of care, 26, 88, 126, 162, 163, 167
Triage (call), 22, 33, 41, 64, 65, 80, 87, 114, 117, 129, 131, 195, 197

Trunk blockage, 46, 51, 227

U
Uniform Call Distributor (UCD), 210, 215

V
Vanity number, 142, 154, 155
Video resources, 84
Virtual communication, 2, 14, 161-167, 230
Virtual encounter, 96, 97, 98, 99
Virtual visit, 2, 97, 161, 164-166
Voicemail, 34, 38, 48, 49, 72, 73, 74, 75, 93, 118, 126, 146, 193, 194, 201, 202-210

W
Warm confirmation, 29
Work process, 25, 44, 50, 62, 93, 109, 110

About the Authors

Elizabeth W. Woodcock, MBA, FACMPE, CPC, founded the Patient Access Symposium® in 2011. Educated at Duke University (BA) and the Wharton School of Business (MBA), Elizabeth has traveled the country as an industry researcher, operations consultant, and expert presenter. As a principal of Woodcock & Associates, Inc., and Woodcock & Walker Consulting, Elizabeth has focused on medical practice operations throughout her career. She served as the director of knowledge management for Physician Practice, Inc., a consultant with the Medical Group Management Association® (MGMA®) Health Care Consulting Group, group practice services administrator at the University of Virginia Health Services Foundation, and a senior associate at the Advisory Board Company.

Elizabeth is a Fellow in the American College of Medical Practice Executives (ACMPE). In addition to co-authoring *Operating Policies and Procedures Manual for Medical Practices* (four editions) and *The Physician Billing Process* (three editions), Elizabeth is the author of *Mastering Patient Flow* (four editions), *Front Office Success*, and *PCMH and PCSP Policies and Procedures Guidebooks*. A frequent contributor to national healthcare publications and a sought-after keynote speaker, she currently resides in Atlanta, Ga., with her husband and three children.

Deborah Walker Keegan, PhD, FACMPE, is a national healthcare business consultant, keynote speaker, and author. Deborah is known for her dynamic, educational, and high-energy presentation style, and her seminars and books are rich with "real-life" case material to enhance learning. They are packed full of tools and techniques that are relevant for today's healthcare environment.

Deborah is President of Medical Practice Dimensions, Inc., and a principal of Woodcock & Walker Consulting. She has co-authored *Rightsizing: Appropriate Staffing for Your Medical Practice*, *The*

Physician Billing Process (three editions), *Physician Compensation Plans: State-of-the-Art Strategies,* and is the author of *Innovative Staffing for the Medical Practice.* Deborah earned her PhD from the Peter F. Drucker Graduate School of Management, her MBA from the Anderson Graduate School of Management at UCLA, and she is a Fellow of the American College of Medical Practice Executives. With rich experience in consulting, education, and industry research, Dr. Keegan brings knowledge, expertise, and solutions to healthcare organizations.

To contact Elizabeth Woodcock or Deborah Walker Keegan, please visit www.elizabethwoodcock.com or www.deborahwalkerkeegan.com.

CPSIA information can be obtained
at www.ICGtesting.com
Printed in the USA
FSHW011258070222
88150FS